#1 Best Tools & Tips from the Trenches Breast Cancer

Heartfelt Advice for Survivors, Family and Friends

by
Mary Olsen Kelly

Published by
Books Beyond Borders LLC

Contents

Cover design by Helen Lindberg
Interior design by Vanessa Perez

ISBN: 978-0-9778946-0-4

Library of Congress Control Number:
2006927368
Printed in the United States of America

The contents of this book are personal, heartfelt tools and tips from breast cancer survivors.
The author and publisher specifically disclaim any responsibility for any liability, loss, or risk, personal or otherwise, that is incurred as a consequence, directly or indirectly, of the use and application of any of the contents of this book. This advice is not meant to replace or conflict with any treatments prescribed by your doctors. As always, before undertaking any new activities or choices, be sure to discuss them with your doctor.

BOOKS BEYOND BORDERS

Published by Books Beyond Borders LLC,
P.O. Box 18696, South Lake Tahoe, CA 96151

Acknowledgements

I have never felt so supported in a project in my life as with this book.

Thank you to all the story contributors. You are gifted writers and I thank you for your generosity and talent; Kathy Cawthon, Barbara Curtis, Pam Arceiro Lanza, Betsy Ludwig, Don Kelly, Pandora Kurth, Katherine Kurtz, Doug Manuel, and Bobbie Probstein.

Accolades to my number-one supporters; my husband and coach, Don Kelly, my sister and publisher, Barbara Curtis, editor Chuck Curtis, all deserve medals for their unflagging energy and love. My amazingly talented cousin, Helen Lindberg, designed our powerful and gorgeous book cover.

Special thanks to family members Janet Whitehead, Homer J. and Joyce Olsen, Bob, Donna and Kyle Olsen, Joan Dennis, Helen, Tom, Vanessa and Ursula Kunhardt, Anne, Arne, Ava and Anson Lindberg, Barbara Le Count, Steve Olsen, Vicki, Steve, Sarah and Kris Kane, all the Kelly's and all the Dennis clan, and dearest friends Diana and Ted Wentworth and Pandora

Kurth, for their loving support during my rigorous medical adventure with breast cancer and during the years of work on this book.

Many thanks to Jennifer Basye Sander for her cogent advice and encouragement in building this book.
To one and all, a big Thank You.

Foreword

I've been pleased to participate in the making of this important guidebook. *#1 Best Tools and Tips from the Trenches of Breast Cancer* fills an important niche; advice from survivors for survivors.

Working as the coordinator of the Katz Cancer Resource Center, I have found that many women are looking for helpful words of encouragement from other breast cancer survivors. They seek advice about coping with medical treatments, preparing oneself for each stage of the journey from diagnosis to recovery.

I appreciate that Books Beyond Borders and author Mary Olsen Kelly have produced this very useful book for patients before, during and after breast cancer treatments. The tools and tips are excellent, and the stories in each chapter bring to life the situations where these tools and tips will be most needed.

— **Anne Lindberg, RN, BSN, OCN,**
Coordinator, Katz Cancer
Resource Center, Dominican
Hospital, Santa Cruz, California

Introduction

The one thing that everyone agrees on is that the earlier you know you have breast cancer, the better your chances of fighting it. The good news is that although more people are getting breast cancer, the survival ratio is higher than ever. Breast cancer is not a death sentence, but it sure is a wake up call.

Helpful, soothing, personal advice and stories from other breast cancer survivors—that's what I wanted when I was going through my nine months of medical treatments for breast cancer. I bought books, searched the web, read countless articles, but I couldn't find the kind of down-to-earth, woman-to-woman information that I needed, except at my breast cancer support groups.

This book was born from a few burning questions: "How can I get through this? Can anyone help me on my journey through breast cancer treatments?"

The *#1 Best Tools and Tips from the Trenches of Breast Cancer* aims to fill the need all cancer patients have: the need to understand "what's next?"

"How do I get through this next part of my path to recovery?" This is the book I looked for and couldn't find. It's loaded with the most useful tools, tips, recipes and household hints from me and other women who have managed to survive this ordeal. In this guidebook, I share the results of my search: information that I voraciously gathered during the year of my medical journey with breast cancer and through the four years since.

The *#1 Best Tools and Tips from the Trenches of Breast Cancer* looks at the personal journey of cancer recovery from a different point of view, giving practical advice from survivors for survivors. The "#1 Best" awards a gold medal to all the survivors who have generously donated their advice, tools and tips on behalf of others diagnosed with breast cancer. It is a reward, a badge of honor to the survivors who shared their best tips with me and for those who are courageously embarking on the scary but survivable journey of breast cancer.

Take this information in small doses or it can be overwhelming. I recommend that you read only the parts that actually pertain to the current stage of your medical journey. There is so much here, don't expect it all to work for you. But there will be a few tips, a few tools that will make a huge difference for you. For me it was the Emla cream. You'll read all about it later, but just know that that one little tip saved me months of dread and suffering.

Here you will find the best techniques for facing surgery, chemotherapy, radiation and the side effects of these treatments. I sincerely hope that these tools and tips will make your way to recovery less painful and frightening.

Each chapter starts with an overall description of the phase of treatment, followed by tools and tips, then an illustrative story and finally a paragraph for the "suggestion boxes" of the medical world and for all survivors called "Wouldn't it be nice..."

The *#1 Best Tools and Tips from the Trenches of Breast Cancer* will be a big help to those diagnosed with breast cancer and their families and friends wishing to learn how to cope with breast cancer and the treatments that seem worse than the disease itself.

1

Diagnosis

"A diagnosis of cancer makes you stop and reconsider, and in that sense it is valuable. I think the art of life is not controlling what happens, but using it."

— Gloria Steinem,
Co-founder Ms. Magazine,
Feminist, 1986 Lumpectomy

Nothing prepares you for the shock of hearing the words, "You have cancer." Before breast cancer, you really don't think about your chances of getting it. Breast cancer is in the news, but it's not my health challenge. I wish I had known that I was at risk. I wish that I had really understood the seriousness of this disease, its epidemic nature. More and more women are getting breast cancer, and younger women are getting it. Like a plague, it runs through thousands of lives. I thought I was protected because,

"My family has no history of breast cancer."

Doesn't matter.

"Because I'm too young, and I'm healthy."

Wrong again.

The truth is, everyone is at risk—absolutely everyone. This disease crosses all nationalities, all ages, and all levels of health. Women and men get breast cancer, people who drink alcohol and those who don't, people who are vegetarians and people who eat meat.

The worst thing is, no one knows why. Or if they do know, they aren't telling. When I was first diagnosed with breast cancer, I asked the surgeon and all the doctors I came in contact with, "What the heck is going on?" They mumbled things about poisons in the environment or the toxins in our food and water. One or two mentioned that although estrogen may not cause breast cancer, it does seem to act as a fertilizer for the growth of breast cancer.

So, once you're diagnosed, you've joined the ranks of millions worldwide. And the numbers are growing. The one thing everyone agreed on is that the earlier you know you have cancer, the better your chances of fighting it.

#1 *Best Tools and Tips*

Diagnosis

1. Biopsy Buddy

Take a friend or loved one with you to hear the results of your biopsy. Whether the results are positive or negative, it's definitely better to have company. This is not something you want to experience alone. Your Buddy can take notes of what the doctor says for you so that you won't miss anything. Go over the notes together afterwards.

2. Knowledge is Power

Research. Use the Internet, but judiciously. There is so much information on the Internet, but most of it does not really apply to you and your case. It can make you even more frightened to read all that's posted. I recommend reading books about breast cancer. There are many good ones available. I wish I had known how to find helpful information easier and faster. I slogged through hours of Internet surfing and read hundreds of books, most of them a waste of time. I recommend Dr. Susan Love's Breast Book by Susan M. Love, MD, with Karen Lindsey. This book is the bible for breast cancer. Dr. Susan Love has covered every possible medical question you might have. She explains cancer, all the choices of treatments, and many other topics in easy to understand language. Other recommended books are listed in the back of this book under Suggested Reading.

3. Take Your Time, Get a Second Opinion, Plan to Survive

Don't feel you have to rush into surgery the next day. Take time to learn about your diagnosis, to have a second or third opinion, and to think and plan. Decide that you are not only going to survive, but thrive. Make the decision to live. Be very clear with yourself.

Say, "I am going to get through this and live a long, healthy life."

4. Phone Tree

Ask one of your close friends or family members to be in charge of calling everyone and letting them know what is going on. It is easier to let someone else do this because you will not have the energy to talk to all the people in your life who will want to know about your diagnosis. Coach the phone tree members to use the complete medical description of your diagnosis. For example, "Mary has been diagnosed with stage one ductal carcinoma, the easiest type to treat." The scientific description states clearly the name and degree of seriousness of the cancer. Then they can move on to answer questions and deal with the concerns of the person being phoned.

5. Breast Cancer Support Groups

The American Cancer Society has a monthly breast cancer support group and so do most breast centers, cancer centers, women's centers, hospitals and medical centers. I strongly urge you to attend these groups. The support and caring that you will find is unlike anything anywhere else. To be in the presence of others who have just gone through what you are facing is powerfully motivational and also comforting. You can't help but think after hearing each one share their story, "If she can do it, so can I."

6. Know Your Pathology and Take Control

Ask for a copy of your pathology report and learn what it means. Have your doctor explain it to you. There will be unfamiliar medical terms, but they describe the type, size, grade, and "fierceness" of your tumor sample. You will find that you will want to read it over as you learn more about your treatments. It's a good idea to refer to it through the course of your medical journey, and even years afterward as new treatments are discovered. Be in charge of your treatment schedule. Don't expect the doctors or nurses to be up to date on your case. They are unbelievably busy. It is up to you to know all about your medical history and to stay on top of appointments and tests.

7. E-Mail Dream Team

Create a group Dream Team on your Internet address book and send an email to all those on the list every time you have news to share. Email is a Godsend because you will not have the time or energy to talk to everyone on the phone, but you can keep them all up to date through regular email communications. I sent a Dream Team email before and after my surgery, as I started each chemo treatment and a few days later to report on how I was feeling. I also sent emails during radiation and as I was completing my nine months of treatment. I loved the comfort and support I received from my email Dream Team and that I could read their responses when I needed them most. I saved them all, put them in my journal, printed them and created a book of the uplifting and often funny emails I received.

9. Happy Book

Create a mini-scrapbook to take with you to all your doctors' appointments and tests. I use a small, hand-bound journal with lines on the pages. Find photos of yourself and loved ones to glue into the front and back cover of the book. These photos should be chosen for their ability to make you smile. I had my infant nephew, my husband, my sister and my best friend, smiling at me alongside photos of my cat. Bring the book with you to all appointments, so that you can write down what the doctors say. It is really important to keep track of their advice and comments, take notes yourself or bring a friend and have them write for you. You will forget what the doctors said otherwise. While you are waiting for the doctor, or for the test, you'll have your book with you to cheer you up. Sometimes the tests are very scary sounding, and the book can do wonders to relax you, to take your mind away to happier places and to make you smile.

10. Call It What It Is

Find out the medical description for your diagnosis and use that description when telling friends and family. For example: "A small ductal carcinoma, caught very early, the most common and easiest to treat." Memorize a short description; practice a few times before you tell people.

11. Dynamind

Easily learned and amazingly effective, the Dynamind Technique (DMT), created by Dr. Serge King, is a practice that gives immediate relief from nausea and anxiety. DMT is a combination of ancient healing techniques organized into one simple, powerful technique that anyone can use.

My husband, Don, wrote the following story, which illustrates the powerful and effective Dynamind technique. I used this technique often during my treatments, mostly to combat fear and anxiety. It worked.

A Second Chance

The technician wasted no time. She looked my wife straight in the eye and said, "It's cancer."

We both sat there in shock. I asked, "Could there be some mistake?"

"No mistake," she said coldly. "It's cancer. It's definitely cancer."

We were paralyzed; our mouths dry, unable to speak for several minutes. Tears made a path down my wife's cheeks.

The surgeon's office had closed early that day so we hadn't yet talked to her doctor. We didn't know the gravity of the diagnosis; we had no details about the size, grade, or seriousness of the cancer.

We went home to bed, and I held her as we both cried. We lay there a long time, holding hands, trying to assimilate the terrifying news. We talked about finances, our will; my wife was picking out her gravestone. Actually, she decided on cremation.

All this torture was unnecessary. Nobody told us that most people survive breast cancer. The technician who delivered the dire message suggested nothing positive, no books, no reading material, and no support groups. Nothing. We were left to our own resources, stumbling in the dark to find out what choices we had.

As we lay there that night we thought, with all the money that goes into research and equipment, wouldn't it have been nice if we had been taken into a comfortable seating area and been greeted by a professional counselor whose job is to convey the news, as well as the many options and choices?

After that first night, having successfully weathered the "knock-out punch," we called our friend and teacher, Dr. Serge King. He let us know us that he had developed a new healing technique called the Dynamind treatment. We flew to see him and had a session right away. He sat across from my wife and asked her if she was having any emotional feelings about her cancer. She couldn't come up with anything, and then suddenly said, "I feel like I'm ruining our wonderful life."

"There's no reason for those feelings of guilt," he said. "Let's get rid of them. The Dynamind treatment can make an incredible difference by releasing stored emotions in the space of a minute. You first acknowledge the problem, you relax the mind, fill the body with breath and energy, and use physical touch to redirect the mind."

He said, "Repeat after me: I'm feeling some guilt about my cancer and that can change. I want that feeling of guilt to change. I want that to go away now."

She repeated what he said.

"Now tap your fingers seven times on the breastbone at the center of the chest, then seven times on the area between your left thumb and index finger, now seven times on the right hand, then seven times on the base of the neck. Now take a deep breath, and tell me on a scale of ten, ten being the worst and one being the least, how are you feeling about the guilt?"

My wife took a deep breath, opened her eyes and said, "It's about a seven."

"OK" he said. "Let's do it again. Take a deep breath, and do it again."

She went through the series again, took a deep breath and said, "It's about a four."

"Well then, let's do it once more." Serge said.

She went through the process one more time and at the end she took a deep breath, and said, "It's gone."

"Do you feel anything else? Sadness or anger at the cancer?"

"A little fear."

"Whenever that comes up, take a deep breath and say, "I'm feeling a little anxiety and that can change. I want that anxiety to change. I want it to go away now.""

We were overjoyed to have something positive and constructive to use in our healing.

As my wife went through numerous scary tests and treatments, this technique was truly helpful and gave her the willpower to overcome her challenges.

When she was feeling nauseous after surgery, she was able to use the technique to overcome it. She went on to use the technique over and over again, through eight rounds of chemotherapy, seven weeks of radiation, hair loss, weight gain from steroids, and difficult side effects.

Glowing with health, her energy returned, we both give thanks for the gifts of this journey. We appreciate every day of our life that we have together. We take nothing for granted. We feel blessed—we've been given a second chance.

—Don Kelly

Wouldn't It Be Nice....

If, when you are told you have cancer, you are sitting in a lovely comfortable room, beautifully decorated with soft lights. The counselor who delivers the news is trained in dealing with the emotional response of the patient, and she or he is also equipped with a copy of the full pathology report and can answer any and all questions that you have. You are assured that you have a great chance of surviving and thriving.

2

Preparing for Your Medical Treatments

"A woman is like a tea bag – you never know how strong she is until she gets into hot water."

—Eleanor Roosevelt

Although you may still be in shock and reeling from the diagnosis, it is time to prepare for your journey. Each person's journey is unique, but we survivors can help you a lot by sharing what has worked for us in the past. In the same way that you prepare when you go on a vacation, you will need to pack and organize your life to take this journey through medical treatments and side effects.

You need to take special care of your teeth before you start this journey, and perhaps get a flu shot or pneumonia shot. If you have children you'll need to find ways to talk to them about cancer. You may need to take time off work, or arrange for babysitters and help for treatment days. You will want to reach out to friends and family. You will want to find helpful books and websites that can teach you about what is happening.

Going through medical treatments for breast cancer is no picnic, but you can do it. It will probably be one of the most difficult years of your life, but in many ways it will be surprisingly rewarding. Look for the good; find the lessons and the gifts. Be open to what this experience will bring to you.

#1 Best Tools and Tips

Preparing for Your Medical Treatments

1. Take Care of Your Mouth

See your dentist and complete all dental work before you start chemo. Your blood count may be too low for dental work during treatments. "The mouth is a mirror for what's going on in your body," says Barbara Riley, Dental Hygienist in South Lake Tahoe, California. She has observed not only that extreme mouth sensitivity and sores often develop during chemotherapy and radiation, but that gum line cavities frequently occur, as well. She offers the following Tools and Tips to help mouth, gums and teeth health while going through chemo and radiation.

SILVER FILLINGS

Talk with your dentist about replacing old silver fillings with white composite to avoid any possibility of deterioration (old silver fillings contain mercury along with other metals).

ELECTRIC TOOTHBRUSH

Start using a good electric toothbrush if you don't already. Find extra soft brushes and brush for a full 2 minutes. Switch to a "sensitive teeth" brand of toothpaste (Sensodyne is recommended).

FLOURIDE GEL

Ask your doctor or dentist for prescription 1.5% natural sodium fluoride gel toothpaste containing Xylitol (Prevident is one brand) and start using it daily well before you begin cancer treatments. Brush your teeth with this toothpaste in the evening and go to bed without rinsing. This helps control the cavities that frequently form along gum lines during chemo and radiation. Your root and tooth structure soak up the fluoride, desensitizing and strengthening them against decay.

2. Get Inoculations

Get a flu shot. Go to your Internist or family doctor and ask for a flu shot. As a chemotherapy patient, you have priority for a shot even if they are running short of supplies. Also ask if you need a pneumonia shot, they last for five years and it is a good idea to have one, just in case.

3. Communicate with Your Children

Children have a few basic fears about your breast cancer that you need to address. "Are you going to die?" "Is it contagious?" "Did I do something wrong?" "Why does your hair have to fall out? Will it grow back?" These are common questions that come up, and the best way to answer is to be truthful, but modify your language to the child's age.

4. Excellent Resources for Children

There are a few wonderful books for helping children understand cancer.

Our Family Has Cancer, Too - by Christine Clifford, University of Minnesota Press

The Year My Mother Was Bald - by Ann Speltz, Magination Press

Sammy's Mommy Has Cancer - by Sherry Kohlenberg, Magination Press

There is a lot of fear and anxiety in this medical journey of breast cancer. The next story shares some of those moments of deepest fear as well as some of the gifts that come from confronting one's own mortality.

My Pact

The middle of the night is the hardest– waking up in a cold sweat. Everyone in the house is asleep and I don't want to wake them. In the quiet darkness, all the fears that are hidden away under my positive, daytime smile emerge.

I mentally pull out my toolbox of healing tips. I do the Dynamind technique and tap away in the dark. As tears stream down my face, I use my arsenal of visualizations. I think of myself healed and healthy again, I see myself in the future, aging gracefully, and doing yoga at 60 at 70 at 80 years old. Over and over, the same sunrise salutation, the same leotard, but the woman is getting older. She's alive, and she's limber and flexible, and she's grateful.

"Please God Goddess Life Force," I pray, "Let me be that old woman. Let me live. I promise I'll make it worth your while."

And I make my pact, I vow to "give back," to pay it forward. I promise to write articles, and blogs, and websites, and books and share knowledge, and reach out to other survivors and bring them hope and inspiration. Through it all, I write like one possessed. I write like a madwoman, crazed with the need to get it all on paper, to write my way into my own healing, to use words to integrate all that I have seen and learned.

Nine months passes and I am done with my treatments. Bald, fat, bloated with steroids and the residue of a thousand chemicals, I emerge into the sunshine, into the love of my husband, family, and friends. Bolstered with Tamoxifin and quarterly appointments, I am set free in the world to survive. And thrive.

One year later, and I'm collecting stories from survivors all over the world for Chicken Soup for the Breast Cancer Survivor's Soul. Four years later that book is being published, and I have invited my talented family to help me in producing the #1 Best Tools and Tips books. My beloved sister is the publisher, my amazing husband is the marketing director, my talented cousin designs the book cover, and other family and friends help out in numerous essential ways to bring the very best practical information gathered from survivors for survivors, all to help ease the journey for others who are newly diagnosed.

I'm experiencing a dream come true – the happy result of a frightened voice in the dead of night, bargaining for life, and now five years later, experiencing the fulfillment of those midnight vows.

Wouldn't it be Nice....

If you could go to a website and share your ideas and insights, blog your thoughts, your favorite tips and tools, and give advice to others who may need to hear exactly what you have to say? Well, you can! Come to our website: 1BestTTT.com and blog on! We want to hear from you, others diagnosed want to hear from you, and most importantly, the therapeutic benefits of writing about your experience are enormous. Writing helps you to accept and integrate what is happening to you, it allows you to delve deeper and find meaning in the experience, and it helps you to feel that you are not alone.

3

Don't do this on Your Own! Asking for Help

"My story should make everyone who doesn't have this disease realize how important it is to support the ones who do."

—Betty Ford,
Former First Lady
1974 modified radical mastectomy

Friends will want to help, family will offer support, and if you are smart you will let them be there for you. One of the biggest gifts of this experience of breast cancer is the awareness that you are not Super Woman or Super Man or Super Mom. You are a person who now learns how to ask for and accept help. Asking for help is one of the biggest lessons for most breast cancer patients.

Friends can help us get through anything. I reached out to my friends, even old friends I hadn't seen in decades, when I went through my treatments. I knew that I needed a support team. I didn't want to face this alone.

My friends were incredible! They wrote cheery emails, sent chemo gifts, changed party plans to wait until I was stronger and could join them. It was amazing. Having breast cancer teaches you what good friends you have, and opens you to making many new friends in your new club of survivors.

Popular singer Melissa Etheridge talks about using all her "Flashlights"—her friends and family members who helped her to shine light into the fearful darkness. We can be flashlights for each other.

#1 Best Tools and Tips

Asking for Help and Giving Help

1. Support

Ask for support in your choice of treatment. Friends or family members may not always agree with your choices, but ask them to support you and your choices anyway. If you want to have alternative treatments along with standard medical procedures, ask them to support your choice. If you want to have the standard protocol and your friends think it is "poison" and pressure you to choose natural healing techniques, remind them that it is your body and your choice. Ask them to please support you and your choices.

2. Communicate

If your friend or family member asks for ways to help, give precise guidelines for how you want to be contacted: by mail, by phone, by email, or maybe not at all on treatment days.

3. Get a subscription to Mamm Magazine.

Mamm is an excellent resource. It is a magazine just for breast cancer and ovarian cancer survivors. Every issue is filled with the latest news in the medical field, and has wonderful articles by and for survivors.

MAMM
54 West 22nd Street, 4th floor
New York, NY 10010
www.Mamm.com

4. Plan a Celebration of Life Trip

Plan a Celebration of Life cruise or trip somewhere you have always wanted to go. You need to have lots of rewards planned for yourself to celebrate your successful healing journey. Once you have finished your chemotherapy and radiation, have a party for yourself or ask a friend to plan a party for you. It is really important to reward yourself for the successful completion of this passage to health. This can be a driving trip, or a cruise, or anything fun and exciting. Make the plans, pay the money and arrange the trips now. Celebrate surviving and thriving.

5. Make Exercise Dates

Ask friends to walk, do yoga, stretch or exercise with you. There is so much evidence that exercise is beneficial for the healing process, even mild exercise like walking a few blocks is helpful. Making walking or yoga dates with your friends will help you to stay motivated and keep moving.

6. Gifts

Ask family and friends to send you a Chemo Gift or Treatment Gift occasionally, nothing expensive, just a card and a little something to remind you that you are loved.

7. Uplifting Messages

Ask your friends to call and leave an uplifting message for you on the phone machine, by email, or to send a funny letter or card.

8. Great Books

Read great books. Borrow them from your friends or the library. You have a lot of time to read while recovering from breast cancer. Beginning a terrific book that really captures your attention can transport you. Read while waiting for doctor's appointments. This really helps you relax and pass the time. Enjoy being carried away into another world as you read. Join a book club and catch up on all the great literature you've been missing. Use this time as an opportunity to reconnect with your favorite authors.

9. Cook

Ask others to cook lots of good food and package it in containers to put in the freezer for later meals. This is more helpful than you can ever imagine. Treatments are exhausting, and it is so nice to have something in the freezer to unthaw and serve yourself or your family.

I am no cook, so I reached out to my younger sister, Barbara, and asked her to come and be with me for surgery. Luckily she is a gourmet cook who took it upon herself to learn all about cancer fighting foods and to fill my freezer with her creations. She shares her research in the story below, as well as some easy and delicious recipes for foods that we could make when she was gone. Various dishes worked the best for me at different times. The soup was wonderful after surgery when I wasn't really very hungry. The African Chicken was soothing and flavorful after chemo treatments. The Chemo Pops were a Godsend when I didn't feel like eating or drinking anything.

Cancer Fighting Foods

Since I was allowed in the kitchen as a child, I've shown my love for the people I care about through cooking. When I learned my sister had been diagnosed with breast cancer, I began to do research into the healing properties of food, particularly healing from the effects of chemotherapy and radiation on the body. I learned about the cancer fighting potential of phytochemicals, substances found in fruits and vegetables that work in a variety of ways to build the immune system and destroy carcinogens in our bodies.

I learned which foods have the most of these cancer-fighting phytochemicals. The ten most phytochemical-rich foods are:

- Cruciferous vegetables like broccoli
- Beans (especially soybeans)
- Berries and cherries
- Onions and garlic
- Carotenoid rich vegetables like carrots and sweet potatoes
- Fish
- Tomatoes
- Mushrooms
- All nuts and seeds (especially flax seeds)
- Green or white tea.

I spent long hours investigating recipes that feature these super foods but that would also prove easy on a chemo- and radiation-damaged constitution. My goal was to fill her freezer with a big variety of healthy microwavable meals.

For Dry Mouth and Sensitive Stomach:
These two soup recipes proved to be easy on the stomach and perfect on surgery days:

Butternut Squash and Apple Soup
2 1/2 lb. butternut squash, halved
2 medium carrots cut into 2 inch lengths
(I don't peel carrots, but you can
if you'd like)
4 tbsp butter
1 medium onion, diced
2 celery stalks, coarsely chopped

1 tart apple (like a Granny Smith) chopped
2 sprigs rosemary
5 cups chicken broth (low sodium)
1/2 cup half and half cream

Preheat oven to 350 degrees. Put squash cut side down along with carrots and sweet potato on a cookie sheet. Bake for about 30 min. or until soft. When cool enough to handle, scoop seeds out of the squash. Scoop the squash flesh into a large bowl along with the other roasted vegetables.

In a large saucepan melt butter over low heat. Add onion, celery, apple and rosemary sprigs and cook gently until very soft and lightly browned (about 40 min.).

Discard rosemary. Stir in broth and roasted vegetables. Simmer for 20 min.

Using an immersion blender or a regular blender, puree soup until smooth.
Add half and half and season to taste. YUM!

Roasted Carrot and Onion Soup
2 lbs carrots cut into 2 inch lengths
1 lb onions, chopped coarsely
2 tbsp olive oil
4 cups low sodium chicken broth

Put carrots and onions in a roasting pan along with the oil. Toss to coat vegetables. Bake at 400 degrees for about 40 minutes, stirring every 15 minutes or so (onions and carrots will look slightly charred on the edges).

Dump vegetables into a soup pot along with the chicken broth. Simmer for about 20 minutes or until vegetable are very soft. Blend with an immersion blender or standard blender. Add a little balsamic vinegar and dried thyme, if you'd like and add water to thin, if necessary. Alternatively you can add about a cup of good orange juice (Odwalla is great) and a tablespoon of fresh grated ginger to the soup instead of vinegar and thyme. I like to serve this with a dollop of whole milk organic yogurt (Nancy's is an excellent brand). Delicious!

For Nausea:
My sister really enjoyed this chicken dish, especially on Chemo days. It was soothing and delicious, encouraging her to eat even though she was a bit nauseous.

African Chicken with Peanut Butter and Sweet Potatoes

1 1/2 lb. boneless chicken breasts, cut into bite size pieces
1 inch piece of fresh ginger, peeled and chopped
1/2 tbsp sweet paprika
1/2 tsp each ground nutmeg, coriander, cinnamon and allspice
2 tbsp oil
1 14 oz. can diced tomatoes (Muir Glen organic are best)
1 onion, chopped
2 cloves garlic, minced
2 cups low sodium chicken stock
1/3 cup or more chunky peanut butter
2 sweet potatoes or yams, peeled and chopped
2 tbsp red wine vinegar

Heat the oil in a large sauté pan and add the onion, garlic and ginger. Cook on medium low heat until the vegetables have softened (about 5 minutes). Add the chicken and turn the heat to medium. Cook until the chicken browns slightly then add the spices and cook until aromatic. Add the chicken broth, peanut butter and tomatoes.

Bring to a boil and then reduce heat so the stew simmers gently for about 30 min., stirring occasionally. Add the vinegar and sweet potatoes and cook until soft, about another 30 minutes. Adjust seasoning and serve (garnish with some chopped parsley if you'd like).

For Mouth Sores and Quenching Thirst:
Below is a recipe that really made a difference during the worst days after chemotherapy when she didn't feel like eating or drinking anything. The fruit and tofu provide both phytochemicals and much needed protein and liquids while the cool Popsicle soothed her sore mouth and settled her stomach.

Chemo Popsicles

One 8-ounce glass fresh squeezed orange juice
1/4 package frozen mangos, or 1 cup frozen berries
1/4 square tofu, medium firmness
One banana
You can add passion fruit juice or other fruit juices to taste.

Put all ingredients into a blender. Blend to liquefy. Add more juice if it's too thick – it should be the thickness of a juice smoothie. Pour the blended mixture into Tupperware or plastic Popsicle molds. These can be found through Tupperware dealers or at many major drug stores or kitchen supply shops.

All the food I made for my sister is gone now. Cooked with love, eaten with love, I truly believe it has made a difference, and I'm just so happy she's all right. Every day she is looking more like herself; her hair has grown back; her body is recovering its shape and she's never looked more beautiful. She's also never been happier. There's nothing like almost losing your life to learn to appreciate each day.

Through her experience, I, too, am living every day with more joy and meaning. Our whole family has finally let loose the collective breaths we had held for the year she was undergoing chemo and radiation treatments. Every event shared is more appreciated now, as we realize how lucky we are to be together and relatively well. And I'm cooking with even more passion and commitment nowadays, convinced that healthy food will help keep my family cancer free. Yet, I know that there is one ingredient that can't be measured: Love.

—Barbara Curtis

Wouldn't It Be Nice....

If all our food was clean and pure, if our water was clean and pure, if our air was pure, and if we didn't have to worry about toxins in everything we ate, drank and breathed.

4

Surgery

"Your first emotion isn't 'am I going to loose my breast?' it's 'am I going to lose my life?'"

—Linda Ellerbee
TV Reporter
1991 Bilateral Mastectomy

Surgery is frightening, but it is also a medical miracle. It was my first time in a hospital, my first surgery. I have always been terrified of shots and needles; I even fainted at the blood test before my wedding.

Once diagnosed you become a medical statistic. A complex pathology report determines your future medical treatments and tests. You are making choices about treatments and surgical procedures that are overwhelming and confusing. You may be scheduled for a radical mastectomy, or a breast-saving lumpectomy. You may be considering reconstructive surgery for after your mastectomy. You will either be an outpatient, or you will spend a night or two in the hospital. The following list of Tools and Tips for entering surgery was gathered from women I've spoken with through the years who wanted to share them with you.

#1 Best Tools and Tips Surgery

1. Surgery Party

Invite a group of women friends over to eat and hang out together. Heck yes, let them bring gifts for you! Have each one write a message and place it in a lovely jar or container. Keep the container by your bed after your surgery. Open the messages while you are recovering from your surgery. Take your time; don't read them all at once. Linger on the thoughts and messages from people who care about you.

2. What to Wear to Same-Day Surgery

Wear comfortable pants, or sweatpants with an elastic waist. On top, wear a loose sturdy blouse or soft jacket that buttons down the front. After surgery, you will be stiff and you want sleeves that your arms can go into easily. Also, you will have at least one drain tube that will need to be attached by safety pin to the armpit of your blouse. Make sure the blouse is roomy enough to hold the drain apparatus.

3. Emla Cream

Ask for Emla or topical numbing cream to be placed on the hand or arm where the IV will be inserted. The cream is lidocaine or prilocaine, a local anesthetic. It is applied twenty minutes to an hour before, and then when the needle is inserted you won't even feel it. This cream is a lifesaver! It can make the IV, blood tests and chemotherapy treatments so much easier. It is stressful and painful to be poked; the numbing cream removes most of the stress. Ask your doctor for a prescription for Emla cream and apply it before you have any blood work done. Cover the area with a "Tagaderm" clear bandage (you can buy them at your pharmacy over the counter) to keep the cream in place. If the cream is wiped off, the numbing effect stops. The cream must stay in place, and the bandage will keep it there. Plastic kitchen wrap taped in place can also keep the Emla in position.

4. Drain

After surgery you will have at least one drain attached to you. The drain, which is a plastic tube, is inserted into your armpit or along your side. The drain collects lymph fluid and some blood into a plastic globe that hangs at the end of the tube. The doctor or nurses will teach you what to do. In general you have to empty the drain every day and write down the amount of fluid that is captured. Luckily I had my wonderful sister with me and she listened and took notes about the drain and its care. The doctor will ask you for this information when you next visit.

5. What to Wear with your Drain

Attach a safety pin to the end of the drain tube and pin it in the inner armpit of a loose-fitting blouse that buttons in front. This is the most comfortable way to be able to move around with the drain doing its job.

6. Ice

Keep ice on the wound area as often as possible. The ice really soothes the pain, and keeps the swelling down. When I left the hospital, the nurse gave me an ice pack. I just kept refilling it with ice over the next few days and found it to be very helpful. Ask for an ice pack when you leave, or buy several at the drugstore.

7. Love Letters

Write secret letters to the people in your life you love or have loved. Tell them all the things you love about them. Keep these a secret, bundle them together and tie with a beautiful ribbon or place them in a pretty box or large envelope to read later, or to distribute to your family and friends if you like.

8. Goodbye Ritual

Create a ritual to honor and acknowledge your breasts. Light a candle, burn a stick of incense, stand in front of a mirror and really look at your breasts. Thank them for the years you have spent together – tell them you will always have good and loving memories of them. Whether you have a lumpectomy or a mastectomy, they will look different after your surgery – and that is O.K. You are still YOU, with or without breasts.

9. You Might Want to Photograph your Breasts

Invite a friend to take a photograph of your breasts. Keep the photo in a secret private place where you can visit it if you wish.

10. Affirmations

Say silently three times a day, "I am feeling good, I am recovering beautifully, I am on the right track." There are some great books about the power of positive affirmations. I've included them in the Resources Section at the end of this book.

11. Strong Positive Images

Choose some scenes from your life that really make you happy. Focus on them while you are being prepped for surgery. It is really helpful to have some thoughts picked out in advance. This will help you to relax and resist feeling fearful or panicky while you're waiting I thought about my husband, visualizing his smiling face, his beautiful body, and his warm love for me. Or I concentrated on my little nephew who is the cutest, happiest baby in the world. I see him smiling and doing his funny laugh, and kicking his chubby, little baby feet in excitement. Between the two of them, they kept me cheered up through the toughest times.

12. Healing Now

Tell your doctors that you appreciate their help and want to actively share in your own recovery. Should you require surgery or treatments ask your medical team to repeat reassuring, positive suggestions...even if you feel awkward requesting it at first. Your inner mind will hear everything, although sedation will blur awareness. Positive statements work very well when your inner mind has no interference from the conscious mind. No kidding, this actually helps. At the very least it reminds your surgical team that you're a person and not just an anesthetized body.

Give each of your health professionals a copy of the healing suggestions. Ask the anesthesiologist to please repeat them as often as possible and add additional positive statements. Make sure you discuss this before the procedure.

It is becoming widely accepted among physicians and health care staff that positive statements can be very helpful during surgery and recovery. My friend Bobbie Probstein wrote a book called *Healing Now* to use when undergoing surgery. Here are a few of her suggestions:

"You will give us a Clear Field"

"You're allowing perfect surgery."

"You're doing fine, keep up the good work!"

"Your healing will begin immediately."

"You have the ability to heal."

Have a surgical team repeat these statements and healing suggestions often to you, plus any others they think might be helpful.

My friend, Pam Arciero, wrote the following story. It shares the heartbreak of hearing of a loved ones cancer diagnosis, and the entire family supporting their mother as she goes through mastectomy surgery.

All the Gifts

The flight is a long one, and I lean my forehead against the cool, soothing window of the plane. I haven't been able to cry yet. The call came a few days ago; Mom has breast cancer and is going to have a mastectomy. I will be there for her, and I need to be there for me, too.

Plane time is strange time; you're in another place and yet somehow, you are nowhere. I let my thoughts wander to a time when I might lose her, not have her loving presence in my life or my children who may never get to know her, and hot tears burn my cheeks

Back at the house, Mom has made my favorite foods. She looks happy and relieved to see me. The next day we see the surgeon. My mother seems to trust him and asks no questions. I like him too, but ask many questions. He answers them all, and we feel that together we're making the right decision. Mastectomy has been the "gold standard" so far, in conjunction with adjunct chemotherapy. We talk about a lumpectomy, but my mother seems more secure with the mastectomy, so the decision is finalized.

A few days later we walk into the Queens Medical Center. My brother and I are joking and teasing her to keep all our spirits up, but the gravity of the situation is etched on our faces. We dissolve into small talk to pass the time; the big talk too painful to say aloud.

I kiss her goodbye as she is wheeled into surgery, and tell her, "I'll see you in a little while." I remind her to hurry up or Jimmy will eat her delicious hospital lunch. She doesn't laugh. I see fear creeping into her face, and sadness too.

Three endless hours pass. Finally the surgeon comes in and tells us everything went fine and she is in recovery, able to see us. She opens her eyes and tears fall. "I didn't think it would hurt so much, Pamela; it's all pain." She squeezes her eyes shut.

Ten days later, we get the first full look at her scar. It is huge. It runs from the middle of her chest, around to her back, stopping just before her shoulder blade. It is red and angry, but the doctor says it will get better and starts to talk about reconstruction. Mom doesn't want to hear it.

"I'm too old, and don't care how I look." She never has the reconstruction, partially because she doesn't want to have to worry about self-exams on the new breast. "I am happy to be alive; I will survive."

Survive she does. I make her a fake boob out of a nerf ball, and eventually convince her to buy a real prosthetic. Her ability to continue and thrive is amazing and inspiring to everyone who knows her.

Fast-forward 18 years and my mother is still going strong at 82. My sister asked her on her 80th birthday how she keeps going. "I feel like that bunny with the drum. You know, I just keep on going."

She is visiting me in Connecticut, and I have a mammogram appointment. I'm running late as usual, and she waits in the car with my two boys, 8 and 12 years old. They have their lunches and "game boys" and since my appointments usually take no more than twenty minutes, I figure it will be fine as always.

In five minutes, I have my mammogram. "Wait a minute, the doctor will be right in to see you."

The technician comes back fifteen minutes later and says, "We need another close-up."

Now I'm waiting in another area; it's been forty minutes, and I'm worried about my kids and mother in the car, and about my boob. The radiologist comes in. "We need to do a sonogram; there is a shadow we can't quite make out."

After the sonogram, and the Doctor looks upset as I try to remain calm. What is bugging him is the fact that he can't find the shadow, whatever that is. They ask me to wait in another room. Then they hand me my X-rays and tell me. "Please call your gynecologist and have her recommend a surgeon.

I walk out to the car. My mother takes one look at me and she knows.

Two weeks later, I'm at the hospital to deal with the lump. This means a surgical biopsy, and I'm being prepped for the biopsy. The only other time I've been in a hospital was to have babies, so it's bizarre to be in for any other reasons.

My husband waits with me; "small talk" again, "big talk" is too painful. Steve has always been there for me, his big blue eyes shining, not always saying anything, but always there. Our marriage is another one of life's gifts to me.

As I'm put on a gurney and wheeled away, he kisses me goodbye and says, "I'll see you later." The anesthesiologist puts something into my IV and everything takes on a dream-like feel. I hear them talking, I hear scissors cutting thread, but it is all so far away. I find myself in the recovery room, no pain, slowly coming back to earth. I go home and wait some more. Mom calls every day but there is still no word. A few more days, and the biopsy is negative; it is a benign lymph node!

At my check up, I see my scar for the first time. It is angry and red, about an inch long, running on the same axis as my mother's. I have a tiny version of her scar, a tiny reminder of our connection. We are bound, my mother and me, by birth and family, by blood and pain, by humor and sorrow, by determination and survival, by love and spirit—all the gifts we share.

And we have the scars to prove it.

—Pam Arciero-Lanza

Wouldn't It Be Nice....

If "Affirmations" were posted on the walls of the recovery rooms and in pre-surgery at the hospital where the surgeons, the nurses, the prep nurse, the anesthesiologist, and the patient and their family could read them before and after surgery.

5

Chemotherapy

"I imagined the chemo drugs were liquid gold. Spiritually, I was very tuned into everything. Cancer got me over unimportant fears like getting old."

— *Olivia Newton-John*
Singer, actress
July 1992 Modified Radical Mastectomy and Chemotherapy

Hearing that you have to go through chemotherapy is almost as scary as hearing that you have cancer. We have all heard horror stories about chemo, the treatment that's worse than the disease, and how you barely survive the harsh medications. Chemotherapy is certainly no picnic, but you can get through it. I got tremendous support from my breast cancer support groups during chemo. It was so helpful for me to hear from other women and find out how they made it through.

When I went through my chemo treatments, it was standard protocol to have eight rounds of chemo, one round every three weeks. Everything changes, the protocol is different now, and there are new and different drugs. Researchers are constantly learning new things and applying them to us through clinical trials and changes in treatment.

The chemotherapy journey seems quite spiritual at times, you are no longer the same, and you are being tested to your core. But know that millions have gone before you and are here enjoying a wonderful life. They made it through chemo, and so can you. Keep your spirits up, surround yourself with positive people who love you, and go for it. Bring it on! You can survive and thrive!

#1 Best Tools and Tips
Chemotherapy

1. Choosing Your Oncologist

Visit several oncologists, interview them, and see if you have a rapport. You will be spending a lot of time with this doctor, make sure you feel comfortable and cared for. Analyze the waiting room; is it clean, well decorated and comfortable? You will spend a lot of time here over the next months and years. My surgeon referred me to a brilliant oncologist, but I realized on the first visit that I didn't like him. He was abrupt with his nurses and cold toward his patients. I told him I was going to look around, and I interviewed several oncologists until I found one that I felt was a real healer. I have never regretted taking the time to find the oncologist that was right for me.

2. Get a Port Catheter

Many women receive their chemo infusions through a port rather than a vein in their arm. The port makes it much easier for the IV to be attached and for the liquid medicine to enter the body. A port will save your veins from collapsing. I had a port installed in my chest on the left side and was grateful for it every time I received my chemo. After you are finished with chemo, the port is removed in the doctor's office, a quick and painless process that was fast and easy.

Be sure to discuss with your surgeon the exact location of the port. Make sure it will be in a location on your chest that doesn't rub against your bra strap.

"PORT PILLOW"

Carry a small pillow with you to place between the shoulder-strap seat belt and your chest. This will keep the belt from rubbing against and irritating the port area while you drive.

3. Chemo Buddies

Make sure to bring a girlfriend with you to each chemo treatment. This will help to relax you and make the treatment easier. A friend will distract you from what you are going through. Together you can laugh and catch up with each other's lives. It doesn't matter what you talk about, as long as it is happy and uplifting. Talk about boyfriends, make-up, children, your favorite movies and songs; just anything to take your mind off where you are and what you're doing. This will be so beneficial! You won't believe what a difference your Buddy will make.

I took my sister with me twice, my mother once, my best girlfriend once, and my dear friend and massage therapist twice, my husband's sister went with me the last time. On each occasion my chemo buddy went with me to see my oncologist first, then we had a little bite to eat at the hospital cafeteria, then on to "healing touch," (a relaxing complimentary treatment described fully in Chapter Thirteen: Now What?) Then to chemo. This proved to be a great schedule, and having a girlfriend there was delightful.

4. Chemo Gifts

Before you start your chemotherapy, go out and buy yourself a gift for every chemo treatment you have scheduled. If you have eight, buy eight gifts. Wrap each gift individually and label it by number. Hide the gifts until it is the day of the first treatment. After your treatment open the first gift. It is really nice to have something special to look forward to on a day that can be challenging.

OR

If you have a friend who asks what she can do for you - suggest that she send you a chemo gift on each day you have a treatment. A dear friend of mine, Jan Amos, invented this idea. She sent me eight beautifully wrapped bath products over the six months I was receiving chemo.

5. Bring a Picnic

Pack some food, bring some drinks, and set up a picnic on the table near your chair. You can eat while receiving chemotherapy. Having some food actually helps to keep your blood pressure from dropping and generally cheers you up. My chemo buddy and I would take all kinds of goodies. We'd offer treats to the chemo nurses, eat, laugh, and have a wonderful time. (Well, as good a time as possible.)

6. Emla Cream

Don't forget to put the Emla cream on the area where you will be poked. If you have a port, put the Emla cream over the entry point of the port, and spread it around the area. If you receive your chemo through your arm, put Emla cream where you think the needle will enter. I'm going to repeat this information about Emla several times in this book because it was so incredibly helpful to me.

7. Anti-Nausea Drugs

There are so many types of anti-nausea drugs these days that you probably won't feel nauseous at all. Yay! If you do feel sick, your oncologist can adjust your dosage and prescribe something that works better for you. There are lots of choices. The one that helped me the most was called Zofran.

DO NOT SKIP DOSES

Make sure to stay right on schedule with your anti-nausea drugs or you will have the unhappy experience of really understanding the meaning of the word nausea. Stay ahead of the pain by making sure you take all pills on time. Set your alarm in the night so that you wake up and take the next pill on time. Don't depend on someone else to wake up and give it to you. Take responsibility for your own pain and nausea management. I had my pills all laid out next to my bed, with a big glass of water, and my alarm set.

8. Water

Drink as much water as you can the day before and the day of your treatment. Before, during and after the drugs are going in through the IV, drink water. The water will flush the chemo through your system quicker and keep you hydrated. I found that there were certain days after chemo treatments when the taste of water was vile. I couldn't drink it. Instead I drank fruit juices, lemonade, and carbonated fruit drinks. After several weeks, water tasted good to me again. Whenever you can tolerate it, drink at least eight to ten glasses of water a day. Put a lemon slice in it to help the taste.

Also, sucking on ice shards is a good way to get liquids when you don't want to drink water.

9. Shave Your Own Head—Bald is Beautiful

HEAD SHAVING RITUAL

A woman asks a group of her friends to her house for a head shaving party. They eat, laugh, celebrate together, and at a certain time in the evening, she sits in the circle of women and asks one of them to shave her head. While she's shaved, each woman tells her the things they love about her. What a powerful experience together.

Even if you don't have your own head-shaving ritual, it's best if you shave your own head. Don't wait for the disease to take your hair. Do it yourself. It will make you feel much more powerful, like you're the boss, not the cancer.

HAIRLESS–EVERYWHERE!

Most women lose their hair after the second round of chemo. You will lose hair everywhere, not just on your head. No more shaving your legs! You lose pubic hair, eyebrows and eyelashes too. The eyelashes were the hardest for me–I really missed them when they were gone. I bought false eyelashes and learned how to put them on, but I never did it. Seemed like too much trouble. The eyelashes grew back in, but it took a long time, years, before they looked full and long like they had before chemo.

HAIR GROWTH

Your hair will begin to grow back about three weeks after your last treatment. Remember this: the hair does grow back. Usually it grows back very different from your normal hair. I have stick straight hair; my new hair came in thick and curly! I was delighted! Unfortunately these beautiful curls grew out and once again I had my own straight hair.

10. Write a Poem or Elegy to your Hair

As my hair began to fall softly on my shoulders, on the ground, on my pillow, I was moved to write a poem about it. I wrote the poem, and emailed it to my family and friends. It captured the feelings I was having far better than anything else I could have said. Write about your feelings in poetry, it will help to process them.

On the Eve of Bald
Feathery Fine, Floating
Wisps in the Wind
Fine as spun silk.

Hair, falling like snow.
Filling downy coverlets
Birds dream of nests so soft.

Angel hair
Shedding like dust
Molting on my shoulders.

Clouds of gray and blond
On the rug, on the pillow
Falling, falling.

Marking the Initiation
She enters the temple
Leaving vanity at its door.

This story is about my discovery of the most useful tip, for me. This one tip made my entire journey through chemotherapy easier. With the help of my wonderful sister and loving husband, I discovered the one piece of information that I really needed to make my cancer treatments bearable.

The Land of Needles

I have always been terrified of needles.I am one of those people who faint at the sight of blood. All my life, every time I had a shot or had blood drawn, I passed out in the doctor's office, even when I went for my blood test to get married. So, I was really worried about all the needles I would have to face during surgery and chemotherapy.

My sister Barbara and my husband Don came with me to surgery. I had scheduled my same-day lumpectomy for first thing in the morning. I felt that if I was really early, there would be fewer chances of my being pushed back by emergencies and delays, and I would get to go home rather than spend the night at the hospital.

All three of us were very nervous. It was 5:30 AM, we hadn't eaten anything, me because I wasn't supposed to, they because there hadn't been time. We arrived at the reception area, courageous but sleepy.

The nurses took me in; Barbara and Don were allowed to come in with me. I was settled into a small cubicle surrounded by medical equipment. A nurse came in to prepare me for the IV. I tried not to look at the long tube attached to the needle that she was preparing to insert in my arm.

Suddenly my sister Barbara said, "What about the numbing cream. I have heard that you can put on something to make the area numb."

The nurse looked at her with surprise.

"Oh, we only give that to babies," she said.

"I'm a baby," I responded.

We all laughed a little bit, but she could see I was serious.

"Oh, all right. I'll be right back."

She came back a few minutes later and applied a white cream to my hand. She placed a clear tape bandage over it.

"It takes a few minutes to go to work. I'll be back."

I shot a triumphant look at my sister and Don.

"Thanks," I breathed a sigh of relief.

We three chatted for about ten minutes, talking about anything except the needles and my surgery. It really helped to have them there with me. I wasn't nervous now, I felt completely loved and supported.

The nurse returned and inserted the IV into the large vein in the back of my hand. Thanks to the cream, I felt nothing. Absolutely nothing. A smile of shock and amazement lit up my face.

"How's that?" She asked.

"Fine, I can't even feel it. Thank you. Thank you so much!"

She smiled, "You know, that was a good idea. I don't know why we don't use it more often." I couldn't stop myself; I jumped up and gave her a hug.

"You will never know how much this meant to me. " I said.

She smiled then stepped aside as the anesthesiologist came in, asked me if I was allergic to anything, and hooked me up to the IV drip. Again, I didn't feel a thing. I smiled and waved to the angel nurse, my sister and my husband. I was wheeled away to the surgery room. My last thought was how loved I am, how kind the nurse was, and total amazement that I felt no fear.

I entered the Land of Needles with no fear. That is a miracle.

Wouldn't It Be Nice....

If wigs and scarves were available for all breast cancer patients to use, for free. Wig Parties could be organized like a Tupperware party and you could try them on with a group of other women. Inevitably this would lead to laughter and fun.

6

Radiation

"This is the first time I've sat and thought about what I really want to do, and what I really want is to be a grandmother."

— Diahann Carroll
Actress,
1998 lumpectomy, radiation

Radiation is usually prescribed after surgery whether or not you have gone through chemotherapy. For me, after chemo, radiation was a piece of cake. It did not hurt at all. My skin got a bit red, but it didn't peel or blister. The hardest thing about radiation is that you have to go every day; for me it was six and a half weeks. It is tiresome to go to the hospital every day but the actual treatment takes only a few minutes. Radiation is required because it prevents any regrowth of cancer cells.

I was shocked by how many people came into the radiology center for treatments. People of all ages and with all kinds of cancer come for radiation on a daily basis. Why are so many people in radiation treatment? Because so many people have cancer—one out of four people in this country are diagnosed with some form of cancer.

Women who decide to do reconstructive breast surgery generally have to wait awhile after radiation treatments because the skin becomes so sensitive. Also, breast tissue generally gets hard after radiation. It sometimes takes months, even years, for the breast tissue to soften again. It took about two years before the tissue in my breast felt soft and normal again. I went to see my radiation oncologist once every three months and she would massage my breast and let me know that it was coming along just fine. This certainly put my mind at ease because I had been afraid that my breast would always remain hard.

#1 Best Tools and Tips

Radiation

1. Healing Visualization

While the radiation is beaming to your breast area, repeat silently, "Thank you for this healing light." Or, if you want it to be more spiritual, "Thank you Lord for these healing rays of divine light." Repeat it over and over until the buzzer stops and the radiation is turned off.

2. Healing Gel Pads

If you have a wounded area from radiation, use RadiaCare Gel Sheets (available at medical supply centers). These gel sheets were developed for management of 1st and 2nd degree burns, and they work very well for radiation burns too.

3. Massage

Schedule regular massages with a trained massage therapist. Massage is one of the best healing techniques, the body responds positively to touch. Massage will relax and restore you. After radiation, my breast was hard. It took over two years before it was soft again; massages helped a lot to speed this process.

4. Aloe Vera Gel

Use Aloe Vera pure gel, found at health food stores, four times a day on your skin. Do not use before radiation, only after treatments. It's soothing to the irritated skin.

5. Healing Audio Tapes and Books

During radiation treatments, you will do a lot of waiting. Every day you will receive treatments, and often the schedule runs late. Bring healing books to read or audiotapes to listen to. Find ways to use this time constructively. Focus on your healing.

6. Cheer Up Others

In the radiation waiting room you will meet many other people, some in much worse shape than you. If you smile at them, and are willing to talk and share "war stories" of your treatment together, it will make you feel better knowing you have helped another.

7. Recognize Your Terrific Odds of Survival

Sometimes, people will tell you horror stories. They somehow feel compelled to tell you about people who have died of breast cancer. DO NOT let this scare you. Far more people live through this disease than die from it.

8. Something in Common

Realize that you now have something in common with Shirley Temple Black, Sheryl Crow, Diahann Carroll, Melissa Etheredge, Kate Jackson, and Olivia Newton John. All have had mastectomies or lumpectomies and radiation.

9. Learn about Alternative and Complimentary Healing Techniques

There are many alternative-healing techniques you can do on your own, such as massage, healing imagery, affirmations, meditation, prayer, journaling and yoga. Complimentary healing techniques include Chinese Medicine, Acupuncture, Huna Healing, Reiki and Healing Touch. Many of these services are approved by insurance companies and are considered helpful to your medical treatments. Research on the Internet, or see the list of suggested books in the Resources section of this book. Be sure to check with your doctor before taking vitamins and herb supplements. Some of them can counteract the medicines your doctors prescribe.

Here's a lovely poem written by Doug Manuel for his wife, Josie:

Radiation
Lux fiat

As children on a bright day
we would hold a magnifying glass
to catch the sun's rays,
focusing the circle of light
on a piece of paper
into one point of intensity,
until the spot
scorched, smoldered,
flamed and burned.

Now machines focus
unseen energy
on those cancer cells
that may have escaped
the surgeon's dissection,
the chemotherapy's poison.

Let there be light.
Let there be life.

—Doug Manuel

Wouldn't It Be Nice....

If there was a selection of creams that had proven to be effective in soothing burns and were handed out free of charge at the Radiation treatment centers? Or even a little counter with products for sale that would sooth and heal after radiation?

7

Reconstruction

"Cancer wakes you up and you say, 'There must be more out there, I wonder what that is.'"

— *Jill Eikenbery*
Actress LA Law
1986 lumpectomy

After surgery, there are options available to completely rebuild breasts and nipples. The Implant and the Tram Flap are two of the most popular types of reconstructive breast surgery after mastectomy. The results of this plastic surgery can be absolutely gorgeous and you might even end up with better-looking breasts than before.

However, reconstruction is very invasive and painful and you want to be absolutely sure that this is an operation that you truly want. Don't be influenced by others; make this decision on your own. After all, you are the one who will have to go through the often-painful journey, and there is no guarantee that you will be happy with the results.

If you opt for a Tram Flap, muscles from either your tummy or your back will be brought to the chest area and breasts will be formed from your own flesh. The Implant option involves a long process of stretching your chest skin to make room for implants to be inserted. I recommend talking to survivors who have experienced reconstruction to find out their views on this subject.

If you've had a lumpectomy you may want to investigate having reconstructive surgery to balance the sizes and shapes of your breasts. You can have breast reduction surgery done on the larger breast, or you can have implants inserted in the smaller side, or in both sides. You can also use a small prosthesis on the lumpectomy side, and balance your breasts that way. It took me five years to find out that prostheses and prosthesis bras are made for lumpectomy survivors as well as mastectomy survivors.

It is your own decision whether or not to opt for reconstructive surgery. You can have the surgery right away, or wait months or even years to decide to have reconstructive surgery.

#1

Best Tools and Tips

Reconstruction

1. Get a second opinion

Visit more than one plastic surgeon and get several opinions about what procedure would be best for you. Ultimately, you will want to choose a doctor who has done hundreds of the same operation that you are considering. Ask to see patients with successful reconstruction surgery. Ask to see patients whose surgery was not successful. Ask to see photos. Never feel shy about asking for a second opinion, it is your body and your decision. Take control of your medical journey and recovery, including this important step.

2. Ask to See Results

Ask to see finished operations, usually your doctor will refer you to another patient and usually they are happy to show you the results of their reconstructive surgery. Ask your friends and people in your support groups for advice. Often the women in your support group will offer to show you their reconstructed breasts as well.

3. Don't Rush

Take your time, read and research, talk to women about their experiences. Look at several successful operations, see more than one plastic surgeon, and then, when you are ready, schedule your surgery.

4. Research Breast Forms

If you've had a mastectomy, you may opt for using a prosthesis instead of plastic surgery. Breast forms, or prostheses, fit into a special pocket built into a mastectomy or lumpectomy bra. Doctors recommend the breast form because the weight of the missing breast will be replaced by the weight of the prosthesis. Adding weight on the surgery side helps your balance, and will help to avoid strain on your back. Medicare and many insurance companies will help pay for prosthesis bras and breast forms. Check with your own insurance company to see what they cover.

If you've had a lumpectomy, one breast will be smaller than the other. This can throw off your posture, and prevent your clothes from fitting properly. There are small silicone "breasts" that can be purchased at the drug store, these can really help restore balance to your figure. Prosthesis bra companies such as Jodee make a smaller lumpectomy prosthesis and bras. For a catalog or more information, contact Jodee at (800) 423-9038

5. What Type of Reconstruction? Get several opinions.

Tram flap? Implant? There are many choices to be made, and it is important that you find a surgeon who has lots of experience with the type of surgery you decide on. Don't just go with a general surgeon for this; find an expert who has done hundreds or thousands of procedures like the one you want.

6. Pain Management

Although I have not had reconstruction, I have read a lot about it and heard from women who have gone through both the Tram Flap and the Implant reconstruction techniques. In both cases, there is considerable pain, and women urged me to mention that you must ask your doctor for adequate pain medication. When selecting your surgeon, be sure to discuss pain management and let them know your preference for minimized pain. Ask for their theory on pain management and make sure you take it into consideration when selecting a surgeon.

7. Nipple Tattoos

The nipple is created after reconstruction, and efforts are made to match the color, shape and size of your areola. I've even heard reports by women who have had this procedure that sensitivity returns to the area! This is good news about the amazing healing and pleasure capabilities of our bodies. However, your new nipple sensitivity may remain the same as the rest of your skin.

8. Take it Easy

It takes time to heal from major surgery of any kind, including breast reconstruction. You should allow several months healing time. I have read reports and been told of significant pain and discomfort during this healing process, but the majority of women with whom I've spoken are so happy with the results that they feel the pain was worth it.

9. Consider Getting a Pet

Pets keep you company, they love you unconditionally, they keep your mind off your aches and pains, and petting them actually releases brain chemicals that make you both feel better. No kidding, there is lots of research on this subject. All forms of surgery include pain, long recovery time, and bed rest. A pet can keep you cheered up during this healing period, and get you outside taking walks again. I know my cat was tremendously supportive to me during my treatments.

10. Enjoy your new breasts!

After all you have been through, you deserve to really enjoy your gorgeous new breasts. And don't be afraid to show them to other women who may want to go through the same surgery. Many survivors report how essential it was for them to see the finished breasts of fellow survivors, and there are lots of funny stories of women showing each other their breasts in strange places.

Here is a story about a recent experience I had that illustrates how long it can take to learn basic information about things like prosthesis bras and breast forms.

Trade Show Angel

As we walked around the Exhibit Hall at the Breast Center Conference, my sister and I were amazed at the warm friendly attitude of everyone there. We easily fell into conversation with nurses, medical directors, and inventors of products to help breast cancer patients. But the friendliest of all were the angels at booth #14.

"Hello, can I tell you about our new prosthesis bras? We have several new designs for our spring line that are feminine and pretty."

"Wow, these really are pretty – not what I expected to see for a mastectomy bra." I said. "How do they work?"

The sales lady demonstrated the inner pockets to us, and even the attachment that could be used to hold drains after surgery.

Summoning my courage I asked "Is there anything for people like me who had a lumpectomy? I am terribly lopsided, a D cup on one side and a B cup on the other. I have just been living with it because I don't want to have any more surgery if I can help it."

"Let me see." She took a close look at me.

"See how they are hanging at different levels? Clothes don't fit right either, they all pull to one side."

"Yes, I see. Don't worry, we deal with this all the time." She bustled around and found a rubbery breast form.

"You do?" I asked in amazement. "Why haven't I ever heard of this? I thought these bras were only for mastectomy people."

"Yes, that's the problem. Most people don't realize that we have lumpectomy sizes too. You're not shy, right?"

With that, she pulled me into the booth and asked me to lift up my top. She slipped a breast form into my bra and stepped back to survey her handiwork.

"Well, that's a start. We can do better with a little more time to fit you."

I was completely dumbfounded, for the first time in over five years I had matching breasts! Needless to say, I ordered several bras and the appropriate breast form and have been gleefully enjoying them every since! I can't believe the difference in the way I feel; I am more balanced, the little "stitch" in my back is gone. I stand up straighter, my breasts are both the same size and at the same level. My clothes fit perfectly. I am a happy camper.

"Jodee" Prosthesis and Bras
(800) 423-9038

Why did I have to find this information on my own? Why didn't my surgeon mention this option? Why did it take me five years to find a simple fix to a problem I had decided I would just have to live with for the rest of my life? Well, what matters is that I finally DID find this solution, and it is my sincerest wish that this information will help you too.

Here is another story, this one about two women who decided not to have reconstruction and were not ashamed of the way their bodies looked after mastectomy. A dear friend of mine who is a well-known author of Fantasy books wrote the following story.

Amazons

As a writer of fantasy, thrillers, and science fiction, parts of my professional life take me into a segment of society not familiar to most readers—the world of historical re-creation, costuming, and science fiction conventions. I've met many remarkable human beings through my associations with such groups, but few have made as lasting an impact as my dear friend Elizabeth—or Catriona, as she was known in those circles.

I first met Cat more than a quarter century ago, both of us just starting out in a historical re-creation group called the Society for Creative Anachronism, which strives to reproduce the Middle Ages in all its (positive) facets: the costumes, the pageantry, the foods, the dances and songs, even the tournaments with their knights in mail and armor. She excelled in many of these areas, but her true forte was costuming. Only her closest friends knew that Lady Cat had already faced and defeated a far more deadly enemy than any faced by warriors on the field: Lady Catriona was a breast cancer survivor.

It was not a circumstance that defined her. As a young woman, she had been a dancer, a military flight nurse, and widowed mother of a beautiful daughter. She spent most of her professional career working as a legal secretary.

But in her off-hours, Cat was to become an extraordinary costumer, not only of historical attire but also of costumes from fantasy and science fiction. (In the late 1970s, she and I both answered an open casting call for extras to appear in the first Star Trek movie, and the backs of both of us appear in the crowd scene on the flight deck. It took me years of searching through tapes of the film to even find myself, much less Cat. But we're there!)

The culminating event that linked her love of costuming with her survivorship was the stunning appearance she made in 1984 in the costume competition of the World Science Fiction Convention in Anaheim, California, before a live audience of several thousand. She had told no one what she planned; her partner-in-crime, another breast cancer survivor, had also kept the secret. I had an advantage that September night, for I was backstage before the event began, waiting to be introduced—I was one of the judges.

My jaw dropped when I spotted them; for the costumes they had chosen to create—and beautifully, to be sure!—were those of Amazon warrior women, with their mastectomy scars boldly bared as badges of courage as well as essential features of their costumes. For those who aren't aware of this historical tradition, the Amazons are said to have amputated a breast so that it didn't interfere with the bowstring.

Even today, it would be a daring thing to do; twenty years ago, it was doubly so. My awed and admiring comment was, "Gutsy ladies!" The audience agreed, and gave them a well-deserved standing ovation. We judges gave them a prize.

It was an example of courage that I'm sure made its impact on the thousands present in the audience that night. I know that it proved an inspiration to at least one other woman with cancer—another costumer who chose to make a statement of defiant courage. Aware that impending chemotherapy would cause her to lose her hair, she not only donated said hair to Locks of Love, which provides wigs to child cancer victims who lose their hair; she then made a feature of her own baldness by adopting a costume that required same: that of a Minbari woman, from the Babylon Five television series. With a gravitas refined from years of playing Queen Victoria for historical re-enactment groups, she was able to lend a like dignity her Minbari attire, including the striking Minbari headdress on her hairless head.

> Lady Cat is gone now—though it was her heart that eventually took her, not her cancer, and at a relatively advanced age—but she was a very brave woman, and I'm proud to have known her and called her my friend.
>
> —Katherine Kurtz

Wouldn't it be Nice....

If the doctors gave you a little pamphlet that clearly told you where to purchase prosthesis for mastectomy and lumpectomy and the bras that hold the prosthesis. It would be so nice if this kind of information was readily available and you didn't have to search high and low for years and years to discover basic useful information.

8

Scars—Accepting Your New Body

"The richness of the human experience would lose something of rewarding joy if there were no limitations to overcome."

—Helen Keller

No human being is perfect. We are made special by our birthmarks, beauty marks, freckles and identifying characteristics. After breast cancer, we have new marks, new scars, that penetrate our physical, mental, emotional and spiritual selves. The experience of breast cancer gently nudges us to accept our flaws, to celebrate the healing powers of our own bodies.

We are uniquely beautiful creations of Mother Nature. We are one of a kind, rare and unique treasures worthy of being sought after and cherished. One of the most profound lessons of breast cancer is self-acceptance.

Life shapes us. Like a sculptor working and molding clay, hammering and polishing metal or carving and sanding wood, the forces of our lives mold and create us. Every experience, success or failure adds to the contours of our being.

Genetic influence stamps out the basic template of who we are, what shape we will grow to be. "Look, she has her mother's nose but those feet are from her dad." Our physical looks; our mental capabilities, artistic talents and ability in sports can be traced to genes from earlier generations in our family. This shared DNA shapes us at the cellular level. At each age and each stage of our lives we find ourselves living inside a changing shape. Our bodies stretch and alter dramatically while growing to adulthood, during pregnancy and with weight fluctuations.

Nature has made us in the incredibly diverse shapes we are, not as carbon copies of a "perfect" body. Now, life has added another unique feature to your body: your scars from surgery. They are a badge of courage, not something to be ashamed of but to be proudly worn.

#1 *Best Tools and Tips*

Scars

1. After Surgery

After your surgeries, after you heal, you will have some new scars. But you will be alive! Celebrate!

2. Celebrate Your Uniqueness
What is unique about you? What can you say about yourself, or what have you heard others say about you that sets you apart? We are all different, unique in our shapes and special in our own manifestations of the physical body and expression. If we could just grasp the truth of this, it could revolutionize the ways we see ourselves.

3. Cherish Your Shape
The concept of shape plagues us. What shape is the right shape? We worry we may not fit the current concept of beauty. Give yourself the self-acceptance and love that you deserve. It is all right to look the way you do. It is all right to be the way you are. In fact, it is perfect.

4. Accept Yourself
As women, we have subjected ourselves to the harshest scrutiny. You can choose to make a pact with yourself right now to end the torture. Give yourself the blessing of self-acceptance. Conduct an inner inventory of your qualities and you will discover that you are essentially a good and deserving person. Bless the good qualities you possess, give thanks for the parts of yourself that you admire and appreciate. You have a long list of positive attributes. If you were to see these same features in another person, you would be proud to know them. Give yourself the same blessing, appreciation, and acknowledgment that you so naturally give to others. Your body does not deserve any more negative thinking. It is time to end it.

5. Shape Shifters

We are shape-shifters. We have all changed shape hundreds of times over the course of our growth. From a tiny egg, to an infant, a toddler, a child we embodied a new shape and size every minute, every day. Think back to when you were four years old until you see an image of your body, your weight, and your shape. Then, see yourself at ten, fifteen, eighteen, twenty-five, thirty-five, forty-five. As you look back, you realize that actually you looked much better than you let yourself feel. If you had just let yourself enjoy that shape and that body, think how much happier you would have been. Why is it so difficult for us to forgive, accept and love ourselves? We drive ourselves to achieve a shape that bears no connection with our genetic make-up.

6. Make Wise Choices

You have a rainbow of choices. We all have the choice to respond, rather than react to the things that confront us in our lives. The choices we make along the journey of our lives will color our destinies. And why not walk this path of life with as much creativity, personality and fun as possible? Life is not drudgery—life is a dance! What if everything in our lives, everything on Earth, everything we encounter is just part of the dance? What if it is all here for our pleasure, our learning and our enjoyment?

7. Practice Enjoyment as a Goal

Enjoy the size you are! Utilize the benefits of your size. If you are petite, celebrate! If you are large, be grand! Maximize the attributes of your size. Appreciate and promote your uniqueness.

8. Nothing and No One is Perfect

Decide right now to change your need for perfection! Nature is not perfect. Nothing is really perfect. Luckily, pleasure and happiness are not dependent on perfection. Celebrate your body, your life, your birthmarks and your scars. Shine your light so bright that you dazzle the world. Focus on the larger picture, the bigger dream, the overwhelming beauty of life rather than the tiny imperceptible details. Place your attention on your contributions, rather than your flaws. Accentuate the positive.

9. Cultivate Self Love

Why is self-acceptance and self-love so difficult for us to achieve? This seems to be the toughest question to answer. It goes so deep, even when we are starting to feel a level of self-love; there are so many layers that remain beyond our grasp. I have worked on self-acceptance for years and years, and I still feel like I have so far to go. To accept one's self, to honor one's own inner beauty and to actually love oneself are the building blocks of confidence and self-esteem. To honor one's self, all self-abusive activities must end. Rather than messages of doubt, we must give ourselves messages that are loving and healing. Once we accept ourselves, we are set free from the tyranny of self-judgment. It is time to be kind to us.

This story shares my "breaking free of judgments" about my new body:

The Hot Springs

"I'm not sure if I'll be able to take my bathing suit off," I say to my husband. "I'll just have to wait and see how I feel when I get there."

We were on our way to Esalen Institute, the famous birthplace of Gestalt humanistic psychology and the icon of the consciousness movement of the '60s and '70s. I had heard about Esalen since I was a teenager, and I had always wanted to visit. I knew about the powerful workshops and seminars that were held there weekly, about the famous authors and therapists who had worked there over the years. I knew all about the fabulous natural hot springs perched on the side of a cliff overlooking the majestic Big Sur coastline. And I knew that it was clothing optional in the hot springs.

Esalen! I was finally going to experience it, on a "day pass." My husband and I were invited to come and enjoy the grounds, see the organic gardens, have a healthy lunch–and we were welcome to use the hot springs baths. Don is a nature boy; he loves to be au naturale. Many times, in countries like Tahiti where it is normal, he has urged me to take off my top. Always I have declined.

Even before breast cancer I was never the clothing optional type. Even when I was young and thin and gorgeous, I didn't like it much. And now, after lumpectomy surgery, gall bladder surgery, and various ports, biopsies and probes, I have a chest covered with scars and boobs of obviously different sizes.

It's been five years since my diagnosis, and in every way I have recovered completely. I've always felt that if you're going to be a warrior woman in life, you'll end up with a few scars. If there are scars from my journey through cancer, so be it. But that didn't mean I had to display them to the world at large.

I brought my book bag (with my one-piece bathing suit tucked inside) as we toured the grounds, had a festive vegetarian lunch, and then headed toward the hot springs. We walked into the large wooden shelter and saw clean rest rooms stacked with colorful towels, rolled and ready for all bathers. We passed an open area where massage therapists were giving clients massages. To the right was the dressing room, really just a series of hooks in the walls and benches under the hooks. The hooks were draped with layers of clothing, shoes and socks resting neatly under the benches.

I saw that everyone was nude and that I would stand out much more with a bathing suit on then if I just went with the flow. We took off our clothes and hung them on hooks. We walked gingery toward the hot springs and eased ourselves into the first one.

There were at least five different baths or small pools, and people were sitting in all of them. The water was hot and smelled slightly of sulfur. We gazed out over the awe-inspiring coastline, the sheer cliffs and rocks of Big Sur. Far below us waves crashed against the cliffs. We closed our eyes and relaxed into the water and let all thoughts drift away.

After a while another woman joined us and we started talking together. She was a Native American whose tribe was originally from the Big Sur area, and she was at Esalen that day to lead a sweat lodge healing ritual. Another woman in the tub was from the Ukraine, and we had the most wonderful talk with those women for the next hour. Finally we separated, fondly bidding the other two farewell. We went into the large group showers next to the baths. Even the showers overlooked the majestic coastline. It was awe-inspiring.

We got dressed and walked back to our car, driving slowly back to our hotel up the road.

"Thank you," I said quietly. "That was a huge breakthrough for me."

"I was really proud of you, honey." He smiled.

"I realized it would be ridiculous to be the only one with a suit on. And once we got in the baths, I just let it all go. And you know what? Nobody looked at me, nobody cared!"

"No, nobody looks at each other," he agreed.

"It was wonderful." I smiled. "I really saw that I am beautiful in my own way, and all those people were beautiful, too. Everyone has their issues and their flaws. So what if I have scars, so what if I have lopsided boobs. I am free of that now. It's over."

We drove along the Pacific Coast Highway, both of us lost in our thoughts, smiling.

Wouldn't It Be Nice....

If our society didn't place such impossible standards on women's beauty? What if everyone was beautiful, all shapes and sizes. What if we all grew up knowing that we were perfect?

9

Be Good to Yourself

"I'd shout it from the mountaintop: a mammogram saved my life!"

— *Kate Jackson,*
Actress

More than ever, during this difficult time of recovery, you deserve to take care of yourself, pamper yourself, and feel like a Queen. This is the time to be good to you. If not now, when?

Most breast cancer survivors discover that they need to give more time and energy to themselves. Learning to say "no" and to control how you spend your time is not selfish; it is essential for your health. Take time for yourself and do the things you have always wanted to do. Travel, spend more time with family, write, paint, and dance.

Whatever it is that excites you and makes you want to get up in the morning, do it! Enjoy your life, especially now that you have come face to face with your own mortality.

#1

Best Tools and Tips

Being Good to Yourself

1. Fabulous Bed

You will be napping and going to bed earlier than usual. Make sure your bed is comfortable, with plenty of pillows to prop you up. This is a great time to spring for new sheets, the high thread count if you can afford them. You will be in bed a lot in the next few months, so make it as pleasurable as possible.

2. Make Love

Yes, why not! Making love will make you feel healthier and more alive! Get that life force energy moving. Changes in your energy level and in your body can effect the way you feel about sex, but if you communicate with your partner, take your time, and relax into a new way of being together, everything should work out fine. I truly believe that sex promotes healing because you are tapping into such powerful, life-affirming energy.

Use Astroglide or K-Y Jelly if you experience vaginal dryness. I've found that these are the best lubricants around. You can find these products in most pharmacies and on the Internet.

3. Eat right

There is growing evidence that the way we eat effects prevention. Learn about the top foods that fight cancer (blueberries, broccoli, tomatoes, green and white tea, red grapes, orange squash, soy, beans) and include them in your daily menu. Try to buy organic foods when possible. Organic fruits and vegetables often taste better and are grown without pesticides (many pesticides are known carcinogens).

4. Baths

A soothing, relaxing bath is great therapy for body and soul. Not too hot, your skin is more sensitive during chemo. Perfumes can irritate, so you might want to avoid fragrant bath oils, but a clean simple bubble bath feels wonderful. Music somehow soothes the soul and sounds even better when you're in the bath.

5. Massages

Getting a weekly or monthly massage will help lift your spirits and soothe your body. Make sure the massage therapist is well trained, licensed, and knowledgeable about working on people going through chemotherapy and radiation.

6. Massage Your Scars

With the flat of your first three fingers, gently rub the underarm areas on both of your arms. Work your way from the under arm to the armpit, to the surgery scars. Rotate in one direction, gently in a circular movement. This will soften scar tissue, move the lymph along so that it doesn't collect in the area, and generally feel great.

7. Arm Lymph Massage

Reach your right arm into the air over your head. Take your left hand and starting at the right hand, gently massage your hand and arm in long gentle strokes, moving toward the armpit. Long gentle strokes, not to hard, will help move the lymph from your extremities back toward your heart to help your circulation.

Switch to the left arm and repeat. I liked doing this while watching TV.

8. Feet and Leg Swelling Relief

Fill an Evian bottle, or plastic juice bottle with ice-cold water and ice. Screw the bottle top on really tight. Place the bottle on the floor and roll your right foot arch, heel, and toes over the bottle for ten minutes. Then roll the left foot for ten minutes. Continue rolling back and forth until the ice melts, then refill the ice and do it again. This helps to soothe tired aching feet, and also brings the swelling down in feet, ankles and knees.

9. Get Your Hair Done

As soon as you have hair, go to a hairdresser and have it colored and styled, even if it is only one half inch long. This will make you feel that you are back with the living, and you'll look better too. There is a good chance your hair will come in with much more gray than before chemo. However, do NOT put Henna on your hair like I did. I thought that since Henna is natural, it would be better than using hair dye. But the henna turned bright clown orange rather than the muted shade of red that was pictured on the box.

Also, Henna coats your hair and that makes it very difficult to color over later. I had to wait for my hair to grow out so the henna could be cut off before I could have my hair professionally colored at a salon.

10. Start a Creative Project
Begin writing a novel, painting a picture, sewing a quilt, or creating a costume trunk for your children or grand children. Start a new project–crafts, artwork, sewing, needlepoint, sculpting, scrapbook making, whatever you like to do–and work on the project during your medical journey, whenever you are feeling good enough. Keep at it, finish it, and then start another. Creativity is life affirming and deeply satisfying. I started writing this book, and worked on it all year long. You could try learning a musical instrument; take a class at the local college.

My dear friend and massage therapist, Pandora, wrote the next story about the importance of massage and taking extra good care of yourself as you go through your medical treatments.

The Rainbow

A rainbow followed me today.

"What a good omen that is," I thought. I had read somewhere that a rainbow symbolized renewal and protection. It set the perfect tone for my journey because I was on my way to administer a healing massage to my friend and client Joni.

A few months back, she was diagnosed with breast cancer. Fortunately, the medical community has finally embraced massage as a complimentary therapy, and it is being done in hospitals across the nation. I was flying in to accompany Joni to her chemo session, to be her "chemo buddy."

When I landed, Joni was waiting, all dressed in pink.

"Joni what a great color on you!" I commented.

She smiled and responded, " Thank you. I like to surround myself in pink because it reminds me of pink skin and good health."

I grinned and replied, " Quick, where do I find some pink massage sheets and pink massage oil?"

The chemotherapy session was first on the agenda, and Joni was prepared. She brought enough food for a picnic and what I call her "magic bag" of healing tools. Things like a reading book packed with affirmations, a favorite song. We were sharing some fruit and nuts when the nurse parted the curtain and brought in the bag of Taxotere. Joni invited her to join us "girls" but we knew she had others to tend to.

As the nurse began pushing the Taxotere into Joni's bloodstream through her port catheter, I reached over and held her hand. We laughed and talked about make-up and clothes and movies, everything except what we were doing at that moment. We ate our picnic and shared it with the Oncology nurses. A few tears were shed, and then, after about an hour, it was time to leave,

I drove Joni back to her loving husband who was waiting at the front door with open arms.

"How is my beautiful angel?" he asked. You could see by the light in his eyes that he meant it.

My massage table was already set up. Quiet music played in the background. Joni laid face down under the sheet, feeling relaxed and safe in her own home surrounded by those who love her.

" I am going to quietly ask for a blessing of healing now. Would you like to voice your intention for the healing you are about to receive?"

"Yes, my intention is for the Taxotere to go directly to the cancer cells and not harm the rest of me," she said.

"Thank you," I replied. " Imagine with every breath we exhale, poison goes out and with every breath we inhale clear, clean oxygen is filling your cells, renewing your body."

I began a combination of Swedish massage and healing touch massage. Both forms of massage are safe and can provide great comfort for breast cancer patients.

Half way through the massage Joni began to cry quietly.

"Are you in pain?" I asked.

"No," she answered.

"Good, then please feel safe to release any feelings you need to let go of, and I will save your place in the land of love and laughter." I reassured her.

I have worked with Joni for a long time, and we have built a wonderful foundation of trust. She felt safe to let go in my presence; she trusted my hands and me.

Ninety minutes later, Joni was almost asleep. Our session ended as it had begun, my hands became still, resting lightly on her head. Our breathing was now in sync and another prayer for healing sent out. I knew we were at the beginning of a long journey. Joni still had a lot of twists and turns and stormy weather ahead on her path.

Joni gave me a big hug and went off to sleep. Hard times were still ahead for her and that I can't fix. But then I remembered that a rainbow followed me today, all the way to Joni's house.

I am sure her storms are about to end.

— Pandora Kurth

Wouldn't It Be Nice....

If the local cancer center or breast center had a community bulletin board with postings of massage therapists, music teachers, language teachers, etc., who would be willing to come to patients homes for instruction.

10

Dealing with Side Effects

"I've had a wonderful time, but this wasn't it."

—Groucho Marx

Nobody tells you much about the side effects—not the doctors, not the nurses. There are some vague medical brochures that list possible side effects, but even other breast cancer survivors are hesitant to tell you because they hope that you will somehow escape the side effects that plagued them.

The truth is, everyone has side effects, some mild, some intense. It depends on each person and their immune system, I suppose. I am including the side effects that I experienced, as well as the ones I've heard about in my support groups. Here is another pitch for support groups—there is something so empowering about meeting a woman who is three months ahead of you on the journey and hearing straight from the horse's mouth what it was like.

So, here goes. This is the top twelve list of side effects. There are others, but these are the most common.

#1 Best Tools and Tips

Dealing with Side Effects

1. Nausea

ANTI-NAUSEA DRUGS

There are so many types of anti-nausea drugs these days that you will probably not feel nauseous. When I went through treatment the best anti-nausea drug was Zofran. They gave it to me at the same time as I received my chemo drugs. It felt like a miracle drug to me because it kept me from feeling too sick or throwing up. I've learned that there are several new and even more effective anti-nausea drugs available now. Be sure to ask your doctor for help with nausea. A drug that works for one may not be as effective for another.

DO NOT SKIP DOSES

Make sure to stay right on schedule with your anti-nausea drugs or you will have the unhappy experience of really understanding the meaning of the word nausea.

2. Low Blood Count

Most people experience a drop in the white blood cell count and have to be injected with Nuepogen or another type of drug that will boost the blood count up again so that it is high enough to withstand another round of chemotherapy. I was able to have the medication and the syringes delivered to my house, and my husband injected me every day for nine days after chemo. (I nicknamed him Dr. Feelgood.) The protocol has changed for this, many patients are injected right at the hospital after their chemo treatments. Lowered blood count is a very common side effect.

3. Inability to Drink Water

Drink as much water as you can the day before and the day of your treatment. Before, during and after the chemo is going in through the IV, drink water. Water will flush the chemo through your system quicker and keep you hydrated.

The problem is that there are some days after chemo treatments when the taste of water will be vile. It will taste like chemicals and tin foil. I couldn't drink it. Instead I drank lemonade, "Sobe" drinks like grapefruit and orange-carrot, or watered-down fruit juices. After several weeks, water tasted good to me again. Whenever you can tolerate it, drink at least eight to ten glasses of clean filtered water a day.

4. Depression

No matter how buoyant you try to be, there will be days when you feel like you're drowning. It's hard to always keep a positive outlook. Reaching out to another person diagnosed with breast cancer can make you feel better about yourself. Once you have been through a treatment, you become a de facto expert and can bring much comfort to another who is facing it. Helping others is one way to deal with depression, but there are many others ways. Starting a new creative project, enrolling in classes, looking ahead to the future, or learning a musical instrument can also help to relieve the blues. It's important to not allow yourself to wallow in depression. Even anger is preferable. If you can't be positive, be angry! Depression can sap your energy and might actually make you feel sicker.

5. Dry Mouth

I found that during treatment my mouth was very dry. Saliva production slows and you need to work to keep your mouth moist. Keep a bottle of water on hand, carry it with you, and use some good chap stick to keep your lips from getting dry. Deanna Maddox Brothers, DDS, of South Lake Tahoe, says that she can read the stresses in her patients' bodies from the condition of their gums and teeth. She described the huge role that saliva plays in maintaining your body's health. Saliva contains good bacteria, which fights infection in the mouth. It also contains enzymes that begin the breakdown of food for healthy digestion. Because chemotherapy and radiation both change the pH and decrease the amount of saliva available in your mouth, patients should try to chew food slowly and completely to help the stomach digest appropriately.

BIOTENE

Many experience dry mouth as a side effect with chemotherapy. Biotene Gel, and antibacterial Biotene Dry Mouth Toothpaste is helpful. Natural enzymes in the Biotene help replace those normally found in saliva. There is also a mouthwash, a moisturizing gel called Oral Balance and a Biotene gum that you can chew to increase saliva flow. Ask your dentist where to find these products in your neighborhood. Or purchase them online at Dentist.com or Drugstore.com.

LEMON DROPS
Many people like to suck on lemon drops or mints while going through their chemo treatments. Sugarless drops and mints are surprisingly tasty. They also help with dry mouth.

6. Mouth Sores
One of the side effects many experience is mouth sores. As soon as you feel mouth sores or painful sensitivity call your physician or dentist! They'll want to stop the mouth sores from spreading or getting worse. There's several different types of numbing agents that may help. One of these numbing agents is sold under the name Xylocaine. This prescription mouth treatment helped me a lot. It is thick, like a gel, and it stays on the sores and numbs them so you can talk and drink water and even eat again. You have to spread it around your mouth with your fingers rather than trying to gargle. It will relieve the pain and let you chew and swallow again.

Radiation and chemotherapy both increase the chances of tooth decay, so you must keep brushing your teeth with a soft toothbrush and flossing gently. Again, ask your dentist or doctor to prescribe an appropriate numbing agent in a jelly or spray if you develop mouth sores or extreme sensitivity. There are several types of medications that both heal the area and numb the rawness so you can eat and swallow again without pain.

BAKING SODA

Rinse your mouth with baking soda and water to neutralize mouth acids, and limit sugary food.

7. Weight Gain

Nobody wants to talk about this, but the sad fact remains that many people gain quite a bit of weight when they go through chemotherapy. The anti-nausea drugs, combined with the steroids that they give you to make you feel better, also make you ravenously hungry, retain water, and make you get fat.

You're supposed to eat, to get nutrients and stay strong and healthy. So you do eat—all day long, and in the middle of the night too. I would get up in the night, starving, and make peanut butter sandwiches and eat big chunks of cheese. I craved fats like this and I felt that I deserved to eat anything I wanted. After all, I was fighting cancer!

Increased appetite and decreased exercise creates a sad state of affairs. I gained 40 pounds during my treatments, and although most of it came off once I was healthy and eating normally and exercising again, I'm still holding on to about 10 pounds or so of extra fat.

So, be prepared. Try to keep exercising. Don't eat too much, and if you're starving and have to eat, try to keep the foods healthful and the portions small.

8. Fear and Stress

Stress taxes your immune system. Our immune system is our only defense against all the diseases, viruses, and harmful bacteria attacking our bodies. The immune system is generally so effective that it wipes out all of the bad bugs that can invade us. However, if that precious immune system fails, we are wide open to disease. Reduce stress in your life. Remove the causes of stress if possible. Exercise, meditate, breathe deep and get massages. Find ways to relax so that your life is balanced and neutralizes stress. Warm baths, soothing music, great books, or books on tape all help to take your mind off your fears.

STRESS RELIEF

I changed the high stress aspects of my career. I chose to focus on the areas of my business that are productive, but less stressful. I signed up for Yoga and weekly massages, and began using meditation and relaxation techniques regularly. I learned how to delegate, and how to say "no."

9. Joint Pain, Leg and Foot Cramps

Many people experience leg cramps and joint pain from chemo treatments and Tamoxafin. To combat leg cramps, be sure to get enough potassium (bananas), and drink extra large quantities of water. Some suggest drinking Tonic Water because it has a little quinine in it, which helps leg cramps.

For joint pain, try massage. Also Ibuprophin helps ease the joint pain. Ben Gay, Biofreesz and Arnica are other remedies that may help.

TINGLING AND NUMB EXTREMITIES
Taxol chemo drugs have the side effect of causing tingling and numbing in the fingers and toes. This is a strange feeling, but it does go away. It took me about two years to completely feel my fingers and toes again. Hang in there, be patient. If these symptoms are too uncomfortable you can ask your doctor to prescribe a medication for neuropathy. I understand that there are a few drugs available that may help.

10. Age Spots
During and after chemotherapy your skin will become very thin. Initially it looks fabulous, as though you've had the most thorough exfoliation of your life. My skin was baby soft for a few months, but as I grew healthier it thickened and I discovered tons of new age spots. The age spots did gradually fade with time, but for a while I had a taste of what my skin will look like in several decades. It gave me a scare, but it went away.

11. Lymphedema
The doctors have put fear into breast cancer patients about the possibility of lymphedema. The fact is that lympedema may not happen right away. It may never happen. I've learned that the number of lymph nodes you've had removed can effect your risk of experiencing lymphedema. As might be

expected, experts in the field say that prevention is the best medicine. There are physical and occupational therapists that specialize in lymphedema prevention. When I was going through treatment they recommended no exercise or lifting of heavy objects with the affected arm. Since then more research has shown that exercise is actually good for the arm and chest area. Ask your doctor to refer you to a lymphedema specialist if you are concerned about swelling. Wearing a specially fitted medical elastic sleeve to prevent swelling of the arm, especially on airplanes, can also be a good idea. Talk to your doctor or physical therapist about obtaining a medical elastic sleeve.

12. Hair Loss

This is the most traumatic side effect for most women. We have so much of our self-esteem and identity associated with our looks, and with our hair. The best way to approach this is with confidence, knowing that although the hair will fall out, it is a sign that the treatments are working. Your hair will grow back. As it's growing back you can have fun with new hairdos. Your hair will look different at each length, and it's a great opportunity to try new looks. Also, there is something freeing about being bald. You're no longer a slave to hair fashion. You save money not using lots of expensive products, not going to the beauty parlor for cuts, weaves, color, etc. You can have fun wearing wigs and scarves and hats. I love the episode of "Sex and the City" where Samantha, having been through chemo for breast cancer, wears a different wig in each scene.

> Of course, it is a huge relief when your hair grows back. Mine came in with tons of body and curls, unlike my normal stick–straight hair. I loved my "chemo hair." Unfortunately it grew out and after about six months my hair returned to its stick–straight norm. Some women say their hair remains curlier than before, some say it becomes straighter. The down side is you'll have to shave your legs again.

The next story is about a lunch I had with a dear friend who felt guilty about not seeing me for the entire year of my treatments. In the story she struggles with her feelings. Many people react with denial, and even terror, to the news of a friend's diagnosis. It is normal. Some friends come forward with helping hands, some just can't. I tried to accept, forgive, and have compassion for whatever reactions my friends experienced.

Ladies' Lunch

Elizabeth started to take a bite of her Greek Salad, then stopped and looked at me, fork hanging in midair. "Look, I'm really sorry. I know I wasn't there for you at all this past year. I feel terrible."

I was Elizabeth's friend, ex-college roommate and now breast cancer survivor. I paused a moment, then reached up and grabbed the hair on the top of my head, lifting it up and all the way off. My head was bald as a ping-pong ball.

"Oh my God," she put her hand to her mouth, and then started to cry. Luckily we were alone, seated in the back booth at the Sunset Grill where it was relatively private.

I put my wig back on and continued eating.

She dabbed at her eyes and reached out to touch my hand.

I smiled and said; "I know it's hard for you. But you have to know, cancer is not contagious!"

We both laughed.

"I know that." She laughed. "I should have been there for you, there's no excuse. I just couldn't deal with it, I'm sorry. I can't believe that nine months have passed. I have been in total denial."

"Look, don't worry about it." I said, taking her hand in mine. "Lots of people have a hard time with this. It's like they think that by being around cancer or even thinking about it, they might increase their chances of getting it."

"I was worried I might lose you." She said. "And I think I was scared that I might get it too. I'm terrified to go for a mammogram in case they find something."

"I went for regular annual mammograms, but I didn't think I was at risk. I couldn't feel the lump. My doctor couldn't feel it either. Thank God for the mammogram, that's what caught it."

"Yeah, I guess you're right." She thought it over as she continued eating.

"I was in total shock when I heard the news I had breast cancer. But at least I caught it early thanks to the mammogram." I continued,

She shuddered. "O.K. O.K. I will go in and get the damn mammogram."

"Good. The earlier the better."

After lunch, we walked together to the parking lot. When we got to her car we hugged for a long time. When we pulled away from each other, we were both in tears.

"I'm really sorry I wasn't there. It's just so scary. I couldn't face it," she said.

"I know. It's OK. I forgive you," I replied, and I meant it.

We both broke down crying again and hugged each other in the parking lot for a long time.

Wouldn't It Be Nice....

If you were assigned an "angel" who would tell you all the stuff you need to know, check up on you, and accompany you to your first support meeting. Actually, some Breast Centers offer Nurse Navigators to guide you through your medical journey. Wouldn't it be nice if every hospital, Women's Center, Breast Center provided Nurse Navigators.

11

Recurrence

"Far away there in the sunshine are my highest aspirations. I may not reach them but I can look up and see their beauty, believe in them, and try to follow them."

—Louisa May Alcott

Every breast cancer survivor shares the same fear—the fear of recurrence. Once we have finished the exhausting nine months of treatment and are set free, we pray that we are "cured," or at least deeply in remission.

And yet, breast cancer recurrence does happen, and people deal with it, battle it, sometimes again and again. These people are my heroes.

Breast cancer may return in the same breast, in the other breast or even in another part of your body. Perhaps a small number of cancer cells survived your initial treatments, or perhaps this is a new cancer. Most recurrences occur in the original site.

While working on the book *Chicken Soup for the Breast Cancer Survivor's*

Soul, I had the honor of reading literally a thousand stories submitted by breast cancer survivors. Some of them wrote of recurrence and fighting the good fight over and over again. Those authors impressed me deeply. They continued to live full lives, they continued to win their personal battle against cancer, and they didn't give up.

And I realized that I would do the same, I would continue to fight for life for as long as I had a life to fight for. This knowledge took away much of my fear of recurrence, I know that if it does come back, I will fight it with everything I've got. And I will win.

#1 Best Tools and Tips Dealing with Recurrence

1. Be Well-Informed

Some studies show that people who are well informed about their illness and treatment are more likely to follow treatment plans and to recover from cancer more quickly.

2. Express your Emotions

You will experience a range of emotions during this medical journey. Express your emotions; it is perfectly natural to be angry, sad, terrified, and hopeful, sometimes all at once. Find a counselor, other cancer patients, or a friend or family member who will be with you while you express your feelings. Talking about your thoughts and feelings helps relieve your fear. Be angry if you must, but try not to stay depressed. Take on a big new project or life-affirming hobby. Channel your emotions toward healing.

3. Let It Go

Don't allow cancer to dominate your life–go on with your life and enjoy it. Here is a good phrase to remember: "I may have cancer, but cancer does not have me."

4. Focus on Wellness

Use your energy to concentrate on getting well, and being well. Stay as healthy as you can as you go through your treatments.

5. Don't Blame Yourself

Cancer can happen to anyone. There is nothing you did or didn't do to cause the recurrence. Be easy on yourself.

6. Find Ways to Relax

Do the things you love to do. Rest, relax, take soothing baths, meditate, read and most of all, just stroll through your favorite path or along the beach. Let the beauty of Mother Nature help you to relax.

7. Be Active

Studies now show that exercise is beneficial to your healing process. Exercise as much as you can, even if it is just taking a walk down your hallway and back. Do a little more each day to regain your strength.

8. Good and Bad Days
Remember that there will be good and bad days, so if you are having a bad day, know that a good one is following right behind it.

9. Garden
Some people find gardening can provide solace and a wonderful sense of renewal. Working with the plants, digging in the dirt, seeing things grow a little each day is a reminder of the glory of life. Let the beauty of nature strengthen you and give you hope.

10. Hobbies
Throw yourself into your hobbies, create, read, build things, paint, do ceramics, play music, spend time doing activities that fill you with pleasure. Plan a time every day to work with things you love. Having a schedule that includes enjoyable events makes the time pass as you go through your medical treatments.

Breast Cancer survivor Kathy Cawthon wrote this wonderful poem. She and her husband Roger were both diagnosed with cancer at the same time. The are both now ten-year survivors and founders of The Cancer Crusade.

The Big "C"

"The Big 'C," I heard someone call it.
Another just whispered the word.

That we don't even dare to say "cancer" out loud
Gives it power it doesn't deserve.

So I'm giving that letter new meaning
And refusing to give in to fear
By reclaiming the power for you and for me
And by saying these words loud and clear:

Let the"C" be for "Cure" and "Compassion."
Let it stand for the "Candles" we light.
And a "Chorus" of voices shouting "You Can!"
To all who will take up this fight.

Let the "C" be for "Cash Contribution"
("Credit" or "Check" will work too).
Let it stand for "Commitment" and "Checkups"
And "Cheer," and the "Children" "Counting" on you.

Let it mean that we know our "Creator"
Is beside us each step of the way,
And remind us to "Call" on His strength and His love
And to "Celebrate" every new day.

To everyone facing this "Challenge,"
I say it's a fight we can win.
Tell all who will listen, that starting today,
The "C" is for "Courage" my friend.
—Kathy Cawthon

Wouldn't It Be Nice....

If there were special support groups for breast cancer survivors experiencing recurrence? Actually, there are. The American Cancer Society has support groups that meet in most cities. Wouldn't it be nice if there were nutritionists who would go over your diet with you and suggest healthier, cancer-fighting foods and give you recipes to prepare them at home?

12

Finding Pearls

"No matter how difficult, it might be a pearl in the making."

—Don Kelly

How does an oyster make a pearl? In my book *Path of the Pearl; Discover Your Treasures Within* (Beyond Words Publishing), I investigate the pearl as a healing metaphor. The pearl oyster takes a life threatening "irritant," such as a little rock or piece of coral, and transforms it into something of great rarity and beauty—a pearl.

We human beings have the same ability. We can manage to take the most difficult challenges of our life and transform them into strength, courage, and healing. These pearls of our experience shape our character, make us more sensitive, more loving, more human, more giving. Often there is a spiritual reward; people find themselves closer to their God after a bout with serious illness.

Look for the pearls from your breast cancer journey. Perhaps your relationship with your career has changed in a positive way, or maybe your family and friends show you how much they love you, or your marriage has gotten stronger and deeper. Here are a few techniques to help you in finding the pearls.

#1

Best Tools and Tips

Finding Pearls

1. Art

Draw a picture of your cancer, and the way you fought it and continue to fight it. Dr. Bernie Seigel shares this technique in his ground–breaking book Love, Medicine and Miracles. I found this technique helpful and enlightening. I drew the chemotherapy drug as Merlin the magician. Merlin was standing tall and powerful, sending spirals of magic into me to find the cancer cells and dissolve them. Others have drawn white knights fighting cancer, or little "pac mans" chomping the cancer.

2. Journal

Just write. Write about your dreams, your thoughts, your memories, and your goals. Write about your feelings, your experiences, and your fears. No matter how many warm hearted friends you have to listen to you, at some point, you realize that your need to express yourself is greater than the tolerance of those who love you. There is only so much that loved ones will be able to hear, and you need to express volumes. For your own sake and theirs, start a healing journal where you can write about anything, no matter how small. This is the place to let it all hang out–no one is going to read it unless you let them. Write about your fears, about your spiritual connection, about what you are going through.

PRIORITIES
How have your priorities changed since your diagnosis of cancer? Write about the things that matter to you, and about the things that don't matter a bit anymore. What will you be doing differently in the future?

DREAMS
What kinds of healing images did you use to help you cope? Some people go into their inner garden or sanctuary; others visit wisdom figures or power animals for advice and guidance. Your dreams may have gotten pretty dramatic during your treatments. Write about them and see if there are hidden messages for you in your dreams.

3. Express Your Love
Let the people in your life know how much you love and appreciate them. Cancer teaches us that all that matters is love. Make sure that those you love know how much you love and appreciate them.

4. Scrapbook
Create a scrapbook of all the cards and letters of support you received while going through treatment. Looking through this book is a powerful reminder of how much you are loved.

5. Get Counseling

It is therapeutic to talk about your experience with a therapist or spiritual counselor. Together you can talk through your healing experience, learn the valuable lessons that any life threatening disease brings, and find the pearls or hidden gifts. You can ask your doctor to refer you to a psychologist, or if you are lucky enough to have a Cancer Center or Breast Center or Women's Center attached to your hospital, they might have counselors on staff.

6. Make Life Changes

What do you hate doing and what do you love? You have had a lot of time to think about your life. What changes will you make, now that you have had a brush with mortality? Adopt new, positive, life-affirming beliefs and practices. You might want to go back to school and get a new degree or certificate. Change jobs or quit your job. Start your own business. Get involved in your children's school activities. Learn to knit, weave, sew, or quilt.

7. Connect with Your Spirituality

Most breast cancer survivors experience a deepening of their spiritual beliefs. The miracle of life is revealed in many ways during the healing journey. As you reconnect with the things that are most important in your life, how will your spiritual priorities shift? Try out different church services if you're not already involved in one church. It's a great way to meet new people and learn what moves them.

8. Moment of Healing

Trust your dreams. Trust your own strength and your will to live. Was there a period of time in your healing process where you knew that you had "turned a corner" and that you were going to be cured? Write about that moment, or draw a picture, make a painting, a collage, an art doll, a sculpture, to commemorate that moment. I knew the distinct moment that my healing happened, I felt myself turn a corner, and I knew from that point on that I was going to be all right. I had a dream of such profound depth that it shook me completely. And it healed me. I write about this experience in the story below.

Bald Women Humming

The wind is blowing; it's early morning, the sun not yet risen. I walk up a hill that's covered with gravestones. Don is beside me, holding my hand tightly as we pick our way between the graves, the moist grassy hillside beneath our feet. We struggle, he helps me, and we keep walking as our breathing becomes labored. Finally, we reach the top of the hill and look around. Far below, the sun is turning the edges of the world faint silver pink, but up here it's still dark.

"What do you want to do, honey," he asks.

I look around, wondering which grave to pick. I see an area that is empty; it's just large enough for two graves sites, side by side.

"This might be good," I say.

We walk over to survey the ground. It looks soft, rich, and full of brown dirt and green grassy life. Earth. Loam. Worms. My own personal compost heap.

"I don't know, I'm thinking that I would rather be cremated," I say, deep in my own thoughts.

He nods, "Yeah. I can see that for me, too."

He takes my hand again, and we walk further over the hill, heading down to the valley below. As we walk, I am aware that others have joined us. I look around and recognize my mother, wearing a white lab coat and carrying test tubes and a Bunsen burner. She is "Science Mom." Beside her is my sister, Barbara. She breaks away and comes to hold my other hand as I walk. To the right I see Diana, my perfect partner, elegant, graceful as an angel; she comes to walk with the four of us.

Beyond her, my dad looks at me with tears in his eyes. "You can do it," he says. "You come from good stock."

But the expression on his face is anything but confident.

My whole Dream Team has arrived. Walking behind me, the group swells to the size of twenty, thirty. And we all walk down the hill in silence.

There is a structure coming into view, a large marble door and a maze of walls looming behind it. To the side is a section of amphitheater seating, and my entire family and friends break away to find seats.

Don holds me tight, "You can do it, honey. I believe in you."

I blink away my tears and answer, "Yes, I can do it. I am a strong woman." My sister and Diana hug me close, blinking back tears of their own. Finally I turn and walk to the door.

The massive door to the labyrinth glides open at my touch. It was expecting me. I walk into the inner courtyard and see a group of women seated on the ground in a circle. Temple Priestesses, I wonder? I walk over to their group, and they turn toward me. They all reach up and grab their own hair, removing their wigs. Every one of them is bald, their faces impassive. Their bearing is strong, powerful and calm.

I sit in the circle, cross-legged.

They begin to hum. I listen, trying to catch the tune. It's a low, resonant hum with discordant minor harmonies. It's beautiful and haunting. I find a note and join in. The humming continues for eternity, it never stops.

But at some point, I rise and walk away from the women, moving toward the maze. I enter past the first marble wall. I walk along the narrow path between two walls about ten feet tall. There is no roof on this maze, but the hallways seem to go on forever.

As I walk, I begin to hear ferocious sounds. I can't distinguish what kind of beast would make these noises. I turn down a corridor, away from the noises. I know I will have to face them soon, but I want to gather my wits, devise a plan, or at least buy myself a little time.

The hallway brightens, and the walls begin to swirl with light. I look at the walls and see a hospital room, with a woman lying all wrapped up in tubes. She is thin and sallow, the tubes have drained all of her life energy, and she is hooked up to a death machine that is sucking her dry. I gaze dispassionately at the scene, knowing that the woman is me.

"No," I say out loud. "I do not accept this." And the scene dissolves.

As I continue walking, a doorway comes into view. I approach the door and am hit with a beam of red light. As I continue, I feel a cool breeze on my scalp and lift my hands to my head. I feel that all my hair is gone, that my head is perfectly smooth. A mirror appears on a wall, and I look at myself. I am alone, hairless. My entire body is bald. Every pocket of fat, every pimple and scar, every part that is out of shape and aging is revealed in stark white harsh light. I look into the mirror, and I take it all in. I see all my faults and imperfections. I see the places my body has suffered. I see my round bare eyes; even eyebrows and eyelashes are gone.

And then I smile. I look into my own eyes, deep within, and I say "Thank you. You are such a blessing. Thank you, body, for carrying me, for serving me all my life, for keeping me going. You have always been there for me, and I appreciate it. I honor you. And I love you."

The mirror suddenly disappears and I am left staring at a marble wall. I turn and continue walking, knowing that it's time to go toward the howling and roaring beast.

I walk faster now, anticipating the encounter with the unknown. I just want to get on with it, get through it, whatever it is.

I break into a run, running faster and faster toward the roaring. It's terrifying, it's deafening and I have to hold my hands over my ears. But I keep moving toward it. The noise is so loud and thick dust chokes me. The walls are splattered with dried blood, with the remains of those who have gone before me. I see the skulls and the arms and legs, ripped from their bodies, strewn along the corridor. But I keep going.

Finally I turn a corner and come face to face with the beast. It's a huge roaring bull, with horns the length of my body. Its massive chest is riddled with bumps and tumors, growing right out of its skin.

I bring myself to look into the eyes. They are red as fire and dripping with yellow ooze. The beast is mad, it's insane, and it's very sick. I see the ravaged form, raging with uncanny power, tearing pieces of life and death and hurling them toward me as the huge creature charges.

I do not run.

I face the beast, my knees flexed. I look down to see that I am completely naked; I have nothing to fight with. I am just meat to this creature–fresh meat.

As the beast charges, I begin to dance. I stretch and move. I glide and turn I leap into the air. I pretend I am an Aikido master, and I gracefully turn and bend, avoiding the charge. Furious, the beast reels around and charges me again. I keep dancing.

I use my arms, making shapes in the air. I roll my head; I lift my leg into an arabesque. The beast roars on, bellowing rage as it comes down on me. I duck under its gigantic chest, rolling on the ground to avoid the flaming hoofs.

It turns to face me again, stamping its hoofs, shaking its head. Smoke is coming out of its nose; it shakes its head to clear the smoke away. I can see that it's in pain; it's hurting, it's angry.

I stand tall and straight, graceful in my body, powerful in my calm.

"I am not afraid of you," I whisper. "You will not win," I say.

"I demand my right to live," I shout.

The beast stands still, confused by my confidence. It stamps the ground less convincingly. Shakes it's head and lets out one blast of bellow.

Then its skin begins to crack open; the meat and bones of the beast fall to each side. The blood of the bull runs thick on the sandy floor; it soaks into the sand in puddles.

Out of the rotting tumorous flesh of the beast steps a figure. It's pale and white, like an undernourished plant. The appendages are jelly, wiggly; its face is a melting mask.

It slithers away from the bull's carcass and oozes toward me.

I stand my ground.

"What do you want from me?" It asks in a voice hollow as a flute.

"I want my life. It's not yet my time," I reply.

"So be it, " the creature sighs. "What else do you want?"

"I want to know your message. I want to learn."

"My message is simple," it intones with hoarse windy wheezes."Live. Don't sell out your dreams. Find the love in your life and cherish it. That's all." And with that, the figure dissolves into a pool of slime.

I turn and walk away, back out the doorway, back through the maze. I turn and twist my way through the hallways, until I emerge from the front door. The stands are filled with cheering friends and family, and then they dissolve. Don holds me in a loving embrace, my sister and best friend Diana around him, all hugging me. Then they dissolve.

I walk over to the group of bald women.

I sit down. I hum.

Wouldn't It Be Nice....

If trained counselors and therapists were on hand to talk to you about healing imagery and dreams. They would listen to you share your dreams and thoughts and help you to interpret them.

13

Now What?

"If you want the rainbow, you gotta put up with the rain."

—Dolly Parton

Once you complete your round of treatments, you are set free. No more daily treatments, weekly check ups, monthly tests. You will be seeing your doctors regularly, but only a few times a year for the first few years, and then once a year after that. You are on your own, and it feels wonderful, but it also feels empty. Many people report feeling "abandoned" and alone after so much medical attention. It is shock to have your life back, and to be considered "cured" even when you still feel so vulnerable.

One promise you may want to make is that when you have made it, when you're a survivor, to reach back and help another just entering the long tunnel. You will be able to make a difference for another by sharing.

I started helping a woman who was beginning chemo treatments just as I was finishing. She had a rough time; chemo really took its toll on her. I wrote her email notes filled with hope and enthusiasm; I wanted her to know she would make it through this challenging time, just like I did.

When I was working on *Chicken Soup for the Breast Cancer Survivor's Soul,* I felt wonderful because I knew I was doing something to help others. And I feel that way about this book, too. By sharing everything I've learned, by cheering on and inspiring others, I am giving back in a way that is extremely fulfilling for me.

On the other hand, you may not want to have anything to do with the world of cancer anymore. Some people don't want to hear stories or be with sick people. That is perfectly O.K., too. It's still important to find some project to keep you from worrying about recurrence or "canceritis" (when every little headache or pimple makes you think you are having a recurrence).

#1

Best Tools and Tips

What Next?

1. Volunteer

There are many organizations looking for volunteers that you can help. Here is a list of some of the best.

RACE FOR THE CURE

The Susan G. Komen organization organizes a race in the fall in most cities. It is the most wonderful experience, as a survivor or as a supporter, to walk or run in this popular race. Do yourself a favor and sign up to participate, or volunteer, or both.

Volunteers work through local chapters and Race for the Cure events to further the Foundations mission of eradicating breast cancer as a life-threatening disease by advancing research, education, screening, and treatment.

The Susan G. Komen Breast Cancer Foundation
5005 LBJ Freeway, Suite 370
Dallas, TX 75244
www.Komen.org

REACH FOR RECOVERY

The American Cancer Society will send a survivor volunteer to your house to talk to you. She will bring a gift bag full of useful goodies like a ball that you squeeze to strengthen your arms and wrist, and you even get a free bra if you want one. Volunteers are survivors themselves and very compassionate; they have gone through a training process and are there to help you. It is wonderful to receive a visit. Call your local ACS office and request a Reach for Recovery visit. Later, you may want to take the training and be a volunteer yourself.

General Information, education and support services including Reach to Recovery, Look Good-Feel Good, Making Strides, and other ACS programs.

American Cancer Society National Call Center
1599 Clifton Road NE
Atlanta, GA 30329-4251
(800) ACS-2345
www.cancer.org

CHEMO ANGELS
This wonderful organization headed by Laura Armstrong, Lance Armstrong's ex-wife, sends letters and gifts to people going through chemotherapy. Participate and know you are brightening someone's otherwise tough day.
www.chemoangels.com

ROAR FOR A CURE
This active organization is responsible for thousands of letters being sent to Washington, D.C., to urge our members of Congress to vote yes for breast cancer research money and programs. Get involved and write!
www. roaringforacure.com.

BE A CANCER COACH
You can coach others going through their breast cancer journey. Check out Lori Misicka's website to see how it's done.
www.Yourcancercoach.com;,
Lori@howtofeelgoodwhenyoufeelbad.com

2. Share Your Story
Tell your story: at breast cancer support groups, to your friends and families, to perfect strangers. You never know when your story might inspire someone to get a mammogram they have been avoiding or inspire them in ways you'll never know about. A woman I know had been diagnosed and she

showed me her port. Two years later, when I was diagnosed and had to get a port, I was not afraid because this generous person had taken the time to show me what it looked like. www.BreastCancer.Org

3. Teach Exercise Classes

Teach an exercise class at the hospital for people in their first year of treatment. There are many easy stretches that are recommended; put together a class that is supportive and empowering.

4. Be a Public Speaker

Talk to groups about breast cancer, about your experience, about interesting and funny anecdotes you have experienced or heard about. Create a speech, tell your story, volunteer at your local women's groups and charities as a speaker. Write to your congressman and become an advocate.

The National Breast Cancer Coalition is a grass roots advocacy group that trains and activates all women and men concerned about this disease to effectively focus the public, scientific community, politicians and the government on increasing funding into the causes and cure for breast cancer, improving women's access to high quality care, and increasing the involvement and influence of women with breast cancer in setting policy.

National Breast Cancer Coalition
1707 L. Street NW Suite 1060
Washington, DC 20036
(202) 296-7477
www.natlbcc.org

5. Hold Fundraisers for Breast Cancer
You can have a dance, a party, a raffle, an auction, a picnic, a garage sale, or whatever you want and create an event! Fund-raising can be fun. Kids give their hair for the cause, kids sell lemonade and cookies for the cause. We adults can do things too.

6. Healing Touch
Healing Touch is a type of soothing energy massage. In Hawaii, where I live, there is a terrific group called "Bosom Buddies" made up of women and men who have studied Healing Touch and volunteer to give it free to breast cancer patients in the first year of treatment. It is the most glorious feeling to receive healing touch—I highly recommend it to deeply relax before you go in for chemo treatments.

The next story is about an angel in my life. Betsy Ludwig was my "Bosom Buddy" when I went through chemo and radiation. She gave me Healing Touch therapy and supported me emotionally and spiritually as I went through my treatments. Here is her moving story:

A "Gift of Healing" Journey

Little did I know that following my breast cancer diagnosis in June 1989 I would go on a fantastic, life-enhancing, journey. It's hard to believe that cancer can be a gift in a person's life. It is in mine, although it didn't happen right away. I had all the shock and fears, and was so afraid I couldn't even pray for myself. I reached out to anyone I thought could help me.

My first call was to "Reach to Recovery" of the American Cancer Society. Next, I called Mitz Aoki, a professor who used to minister to those with life threatening illnesses. Through prayer and guided imagery, he turned my focus away from fear and brought me to look into our Lord's face and see peace within me, and see myself healing.

I created a team of loving people and a healing environment around me, medically, spiritually, emotionally and physically. Bernie Siegel, in his book, Love, Medicine and Miracles, calls these people "Exceptional Cancer Patients." He says we can't rely only on the doctor to help us; we play a major part in our own healing. What began to happen to me was a feeling that I could be in control of my life again, a feeling I thought I had lost.

I began to "journal" during these times. I wrote down all the scary stuff, the frustrations, and the mountaintop and valley experiences. It meant so much to reread my journal days later to see where I had been and how far I had come.

I found a cancer support group at a local church led by a woman who was recovering from breast cancer. She, too, used guided imagery that she had composed. She took us, in our imagination, to places where we could feel comfortable, peaceful and safe: on a beach chair by the ocean, in a flowering garden, beside a gentle, trickling stream. We left feeling relaxed, refreshed and restored.

The cancer support group became a part of my life, and our leader asked me to take over the group when her breast cancer recurred. Creating my own meditations and prayers and sharing them with others was where I wanted and needed to be. At that point, I realized my healing journey had become a "gift" to me. I continued to have my eyes open for other ways to share my "gift" on my healing journey.

In 1996, I took a class on "energy centers" of the body that was offered for interested volunteers at Queen's Medical Center. It is called "Healing Touch," as it is a "hands on" type of complimentary medicine. I asked to volunteer in the Radiation Therapy Department so I could be there for cancer patients. I see the patients in the waiting room, their faces full of concern, and invite them to have Healing Touch in a room where we have a bed set aside. I play soft music and pray silently, or aloud, whichever the person prefers. I show how to relax body and mind, and by placing my hand over the energy centers, bring mind, body and spirit back into peace, harmony, and wellness.

I began to introduce guided imagery into our sessions. Several patients wished they could have a private cassette tape of our sessions. I asked them in their imagination to go to a special place of their own, using all their senses and describe the scene to me. I wrote down all their words. The tape began with relaxation, and then I repeated back to them the thoughts and the scene they had chosen, along with reinforcing, healing words. Their faces became peaceful, sometimes with a gentle smile. One patient went to her favorite childhood park to swing higher and higher; another to a vacation on the beach in Bali with warm trade winds; another to hang gliding over a beach, soaring for two hours. They were really there, no doubt in my mind. Energetic, but peaceful, with a sense of well being that their bodies acknowledged and responded by healing.

I became a participant in the Bosom Buddies program under Healing Touch about four years ago. We adopt a breast cancer patient and serve her for six months in any way we can. I have had four Bosom Buddies and my first was an exceptional cancer patient. She always had a notebook with her at our sessions and said she was an author and wanted to write a book. I'm sure she has.

My latest quest has been to create and record a CD of "Relaxation and Guided Imagery" for all patients in our department and any other hospital patient who wants one. Our patients are well on their way into their healing journey as we provide them with healing tools to help themselves—a respite in times of need.

We are here on earth to love each other and to take care of each other. I'm deeply honored to share my "gift of healing" wherever I can. I am truly blessed.

—Betsy Ludwig

Wouldn't It Be Nice....

To have "Healing Touch" practitioners available at every hospital, free of charge to people having surgery and going through chemotherapy and radiation.

14

How Can Friends and Family Offer Support

"Difficult times have helped me to understand better than before how infinitely rich and beautiful life is..."

—Isak Dinesen

If there was ever a time in your life that you needed friends and family, this is it. Suddenly all that matters is the people you love and the people who love you back. Everything else pales by comparison, and you feel your priorities line up pretty clearly. I reached out to my friends and family and they were right there for me. I suggest that you do the same—hold out your hand and ask for help. They will be there, in spades.

#1

Best Tools and Tips

How Friends Can Offer Support

1. Biopsy, Chemo, Radiation Buddies

Go with your friend to the biopsy, go to the chemo treatments as a Chemo Buddy, go to the radiation treatments. It is tremendously supportive to have someone with you when you go through scary tests and treatments. Call and ask when the next treatment is and see if you can go, too.

2. Cooking for the Freezer

Yes, yes yes. This can't be overemphasized–food is love! Create healthy dishes that can be stored and frozen for later. Make lasagna, or a chicken dish, or your favorite brown rice casserole. Soup is fabulous too unthaw later. Make healthful, tasty (but not spicy) dishes and store them in freezer containers for later use. Tupperware makes great sizes and shapes, you can make a dinner for one, or two, or four, or ten using the different sizes Tupperware freezer containers.

3. Form a Communication Team

PHONE DIRECTOR

Assign a phone director, just one person, to be in charge of phoning family members.

PHONE TREE

It works well to choose one person from each branch of family or friends, and ask that person to call the others. That way, everyone will know how the patient is doing, without you having to face the overwhelming task of lots of phone calls.

CREATE AN EMAIL DREAM TEAM FOR YOUR FRIENDS AND FAMILY

Make an email address list of all family and friends who will want to know about your friend's progress. She will not feel like talking to all of them on the phone, the email allows her to stay in contact with everybody, lets her know how much she matters to you as you send prayers, healing energy, jokes, inspirational quotes, cheerful remarks, and personal news. It is so wonderful to receive uplifting cheerful messages from friends and family. A simple "How are you doing? Just thinking of you." Is all that's needed–if your friend feels up to responding, she can on her own time. Stay in touch in a soft, sensitive, respectful way. Tune in to their needs, knowing that your friend may not have the energy to call you right back. Make sure to say "No need to call me back, I just want you to know I'm thinking of you."

4. Wig Shopping

Go out to several wig stores and have a blast trying on lots of wigs. Wigs are all different colors and styles, and they can be really quite flattering. Have fun with all the different sides to your personality! My best friend and I went wig shopping and laughed constantly. It was such fun; we both remember it as one of the funniest days we have ever shared. And it made a huge difference to me to have someone I love help me find a flattering wig for the bald days to come.

5. Ladies Lunch

Get some friends together and take your friend to lunch at a great spot! Dress up, wear hats, have fun. Talk about clothes and men and make-up and anything and everything except cancer. Assume survival, and total health. Act "as if" she is already cured and all this is behind her. Because it will be, soon. Don't offer advice or commiserate, just have fun together like nothing was wrong.

6. Walking Together

There's so much evidence about the benefits of walking while recovering from treatments. Grab your walking shoes and your friend and get out there! Make walking dates, around a lake, around a park, through the city. Walk and talk and laugh and sweat.

7. Scary Test Gifts

Find out chemo dates, radiation dates, dates for MRIs and send a little gift in the mail or leave it on the doorstep on scary test days. Thoughtfulness like this is precious and will never be forgotten.

8. Chemo Gifts

Buy a small gift for each round of chemo. Send it or give it in person to commemorate that another round of treatments is over. Hallelujah!

9. Listen

Let them cry, or talk, or rage, or whine. Offer support and a good listening ear. Say things like "This is the pits. I think you have every right to be angry at the cancer." Talk about other things, not just the diagnosis, when you're together. Share the little details of your life, the things happening at work. Act as normal as possible. Affirm health and survival. But don't be hesitant to talk about the medical journey also. Be natural, be curious, and be there.

10. Talk talk talk talk talk

Talk and listen and talk some more. Talking about feelings is healing. Talk about dreams, goals, fears, and hurts. Just talk about everything. Support their choices of treatment, medical as well as alternative and complimentary treatments. Until you are hearing the words, "You have cancer," yourself, you don't know how you would respond. Honor the choices they make and support them in their journey.

11. Help with the kids, the grocery shopping, and the bill paying

Duh. This is so obvious it hardly needs to be included, but in case you didn't think of these basic things, here they are. Grocery shopping is tiring, bill paying takes focus, and the kids have their own needs and schedules. Helping with any of these things will be appreciated.

This beautiful story by my friend, Bobbie Probstein, illustrates the poignancy and love we feel for a friend who is battling breast cancer.

Friends

Anna had always drawn others to her like a magnet because of her bubbly, warm personality, sincere interest in people and her outstretched hand of friendship. We lived far apart now and that had cut back on our adventures, if not the long distance calls.

We sat in the park under a shady tree and reminisced about old times, good times. We had known each other for more than thirty years, and talked about our grown children, work, school and double-dating way back in college. But sometimes what isn't said is as important as what is said, and Anna didn't mention her husband, soon to be an ex.

She spoke about her recent diagnosis of breast cancer, and how her employer, an international company, had understood the need for some time off and kept her on their payroll. Cancer support groups and a large circle of friends had helped enormously to keep her spirits up in spite of the rounds of treatments she was undergoing. Anna said, "I envision the drips in my arm as being white knights, jousting with the germs and winning the battle," but changed the subject quickly.

Then she started to giggle. "I had a dream the other night. Remember, about five years ago, when we decided to ride a merry-go-round and be like kids again?"

"Oh, yes! That was fun. I always loved riding horses," and I began to giggle too, recalling how our plan had been to spend the day with no adult concerns or discussions.

"Well," she said, "In the dream, I was on this white horse, holding on to the pole, going up and down and up and down, and loving it...tinny, repetitious music that never seems to stop. I wanted to just fly away on the horse, into the sky, away from the pole and the music—away from everything that held me down. I imagined myself above the earth, a starry sky above me, the big white horse galloping freely and his mane blowing in the wind, and I was free—free and full of joy again!"

"What a wonderful image!" I said, hugging her, keeping my arms around my friend just a little longer than usual.

—Bobbie Probstein

#1 Best Tools and Tips

How Family Can Offer Support

1. Stop Working So Much

Once a partner has been diagnosed with breast cancer, many couples realize that work has been the focus of their lives. Cancer teaches one profound lesson–that life is short. Take time with your loved ones, travel, follow your passions, and create a balanced life.

2. Spend Time Together

Create reasons to spend time with family members, sisters, brothers, parents, cousins, and grandparents, if you are lucky enough to have them. Just be together, have barbecues, take a cruise together, take walks together. Whatever the cancer patient feels like doing, just sharing time together is precious.

3. Read Out Loud to Each Other

Before TV, people used to read out loud to each other, recite poems, and stage plays. Reading out loud is entertaining, educational, and includes the whole family. Trade off reading, pass the book around and each person takes a page or two.

4. Learn a Musical Instrument Together

Ever wanted to play piano? Violin? Mandolin? Now is the time; learn to play a musical instrument and practice a piece to perform for your friends and family. Learning music stimulates your brain, keeps you young at heart, and feeds the soul, and will probably keep your family member with cancer vastly amused. Why not start a family band?

5. Learn a New Language Together

Learning a language is exercise for the brain, keeping you young and healthy, mentally alert and alive. Learn Spanish, or French, and practice by planning to take a trip to that country when the family member with cancer has recovered from her treatments. Practice on everybody—make a fool of yourself. Who cares? Dive in and try it.

6. Travel as a Family

My family has taken many trips together, and it is sheer pleasure for all of us. We love cruise ships, because everybody has their own room, their own agenda during the day, and then we join together for dinner every night and share our day's activities. This is one of the most enjoyable ways to be together as a family; try it!

7. Old Fashioned Family Entertainment

How about charades? Put on a skit? Sing a song, perform a dance routine, perform with your musical instrument. Have holiday parties, Halloween, May Day, Mother's Day, and use the holiday as a theme for performances. This is something my family has been doing for a decade, and it is something we all plan for and look forward to. Costumes, sets, the works go into short little skits and songs. We videotape the event and the kids watch it over and over, year after year.

8. Listen to Experts on Tape Together

Audiotapes by doctors and breast cancer specialists are great to listen to while waiting for doctors, relaxing at home, or driving in your car. There are some wonderfully informative books on tape about healing, meditation, and visualization as well. But my very favorites were from the Healing Journeys Conferences.

In this tape set, called "Cancer as a Turning Point," breast cancer survivors, authors, psychologists and doctors shared personal and uplifting messages of hope. These speakers inspired me tremendously.

FAVORITE TAPES:

Dr. Bernie S. Siegel, *Love Medicine and Miracles,* Harper Audio

Healing Journeys, Cancer as a Turning Point, Sounds True Audio

Dr. Carl Simonton, *Getting Well,* Audio Renaissance Tapes

9. Create a Family Quilt

Have each family member create a square; they can use their own fabrics, designs, even write a saying on their square. Then, at a family gathering, lay out all the squares and sew the quilt together. Then it can be hung in a place of honor.

10. Create Your Legacy

What are you leaving behind for your children and grandchildren? Make a family scrapbook with highlights, create a family tree, study your genealogy, write a book about all the family stories and memories.

Here is a story about the way my mother reacted when I told her I had been diagnosed with breast cancer:

Science Mom

Telling people I had Breast Cancer was one of the hardest parts. Why? Because I was afraid of their reaction—that it would weaken me, that we would both cry, that we would fall apart. I was most worried to tell my parents.

Luckily, Ted, a wise friend who had been through the journey before, guided me. He had lost his first wife to cancer, and was well versed in the strange and separate world that one enters after hearing the words: "You have cancer."

"Keep it simple," he said. "Stick to the facts."

He urged me to find out the exact medical terminology for my type of cancer, and use those terms when describing it to people for the first time. "If it's 'a small ductal carcinoma, the easiest type to treat,' then that's what you should say."

I practiced saying it a few times until it rolled off my tongue easily, and then called my family.

I called my Mother this morning and was very worried about what her reaction might be. I didn't want to scare her.

"Hi Mother, I have some news about my recent mammogram I need to tell you. They found a small ductal carcinoma, the easiest type to treat, and with the best success rates."

I waited for her terrified response. To my utter shock, her reaction was quite the opposite—she was wonderful. She just listened, and then asked intelligent questions, and then more questions about the scientific aspects. She became "science mom." It was great.

I don't know what I thought—she has always been strong in crises, and I felt really confident after talking to her. I told her it would be OK to tell everyone—in fact, I would welcome it. My fear of telling others turned out to be nonsense, because everybody has been fantastic and very strong and calm.

But I know that Ted's advice made it possible for all of us to pass through this frightening phase of the emotional and medical journey of breast cancer. Knowledge is power, and the ability to simplify and understand the enemy made it easier for me, my family, and my friends, to deal with it. He gave the fear a name, and when something has a name it is robbed of its power.

Wouldn't It Be Nice....

If we didn't have to get sick to remember the basics of living a good life. Cancer sets your priorities straight. You get very clear about what really matters in life. To me, the most important thing in life is love; the love you give, and the love you receive from those who love you back.

15

The Road Back to Health

"We all have big changes in our lives that are more or less a second chance."

—Harrison Ford

Congratulations, you are finished with treatments. You are on the mend! Each day you will feel better and you will be reminded of the miracle of your healing body. After one year, I thought I was completely 100 percent. After two years, I realized that I was back much more, and, after three and four years, I continued to feel stronger. At five years, I am convinced that I am 1,000 percent back to my old self: healthy, full of energy, pain-free. But who knows, maybe in another year or so I'll feel even better! That is the miracle of the healing process—it is subtle and gradual and then, all of a sudden, you realize you feel much better.

Many people experience profound transformation after breast cancer. For many survivors, the disease is almost considered to be a gift. There are so many gifts that come from serious disease–spiritual changes, physical lifestyle changes, relationship changes, and priority changes. It is a huge wake-up call and an opportunity to change your life profoundly.

#1 Best Tools and Tips

The Road Back to Health

1. Lifestyle Changes

Your life has been shuffled; your priorities have changed. Put the changes into action. If you want to change jobs or retire, do it. If you want to spend more time in nature, with your family or writing your novel, do it. Life has given you a second chance. Take the chance.

2. Dietary Changes

Breast cancer survivors often switch to being vegetarians, or at least putting more emphasis on eating cancer-fighting foods. Vitamins and supplements become more important as we continue our fight against recurrence by building up our immune systems. Organic foods, clean filtered water, vitamins, diligently using sunscreen, switching to organic deodorant, natural make-up and water–based nail polish are all good ideas.

3. Deodorant

Although there are no clinical tests to prove this, many women feel better changing from antiperspirant to "all natural" deodorant after breast cancer. Many deodorants and antiperspirants contain chemicals that may cause irritation or be harmful to your body. Deodorants from the health food store usually don't contain heavy metals that can be toxic or even carcinogenic. There are many great brands, such as Tom's. I found myself switching to Tom's deodorant, as well as Tom's toothpaste and mouthwash. It just felt better to be using grooming products containing ingredients that weren't potentially harmful to my newly healed body.

4. Hot Flashes

If you're required, like I was, to take Tamoxifin for years following your treatments, you'll be thrust into menopause and hot flashes. You can try experimenting with natural herbs that may help hot flashes, like black cohash and wild yam extract. Unfortunately, no matter what you try, you will probably have to just tough it out and fling the covers off during the night like the rest of us. Oddly, there is substantial evidence that low doses of prescription anti-depressants like Paxil and Prozac actually relieve hot flashes (or "flushing" as the medical world calls it). If your menopausal symptoms are too unpleasant, try discussing these options with your doctor.

5. Energy Level

Fatigue and low energy can be difficult problems after treatments. The best thing to do is take a nap. Naps in the afternoon are restorative and regenerative. Or, take a bath and relax. Low energy level could be one way your body is telling you to relax and heal.

6. Underwires

The underwires in bras are a subject of much debate among survivors. It is thought that the wires can inhibit circulation and this might compromise the healthy function of breast cells. Anything that cuts off blood flow and oxygen might increase the risk. There is no medical proof for this, but it made sense to me, so I took all the underwires out of my bras. They work just as well without them, and I just feel better not having any extra deterrent to circulation.

7. Sex, Intimacy and Love

Some women report feeling diminished sexual drive, vaginal dryness, sensitivity, and discomfort during and even after treatments. Often, their partners feel shy about approaching the survivor to initiate lovemaking, fearing that they will cause them additional pain. This is such a personal thing; it is different for each of us. The best solution is to communicate with your partner, talk about your areas of sensitivity, and agree to proceed gently and slowly. Holding each other, cuddling, being sexually playful, and touching can provide feelings of sexual closeness without actual penetration. Your recovery can be a time to connect on an even deeper level than before, to get close, beyond the surface, so that you feel you are connecting on a soul level. Sex, when you're ready, can then bring your love for each other to an even closer, more caring and connected place. I thought that I loved my husband as much as one human being could love another. Breast cancer taught me that there was even more love to give and to receive–it made both of us fall even more deeply in love.

8. Humor

Laughter really is the best medicine. Try to find the humor in your life, in your medical journey, and in your recovery. There are even studies that have found that laughter stimulates the immune system and is beneficial in healing. So laugh away! See funny movies, collect jokes from friends, watch comedy on TV or in the comedy clubs. Enjoy!

9. Attitude

I know you've heard this a lot from me, but it is a fact: A positive attitude is helpful. There are even theories that your attitude influences your immune system. Sure, sometimes you don't feel like it. But, keep your thoughts positive and you will feel better in general. Look for the "gift" in everything, collect the pearls from your experiences. Your life is a precious evolving story. Make it a happy, positive, and loving story.

10. Path of the Pearl

The pearl oyster transforms potentially fatal irritants into gems of great rarity and beauty. How can we take the challenges of our lives and turn them into pearls of strength, healing and beauty?

I wrote the next story for my sister. I am so blessed to have the most wonderful, loving, supportive sister. As we've gotten older, we've become closer. She is even supporting me in this book project: she is my publisher! In fact, the entire book is a family project. It seems everyone in the family is pitching in to help, and that is another gift of having breast cancer. It has brought us all closer together. For that I am deeply grateful.

The Olsen Girls

My little sister turned fifty today—the one I carried around, she: one-year- old, me: two-and-a-half. I told everyone, "My baby. This is my baby."

She of the naturally curly blond ponytail and big blue eyes, "Oh, she looks like a princess," strangers would exclaim. My brown eyes downcast, I nodded, straight brown hair bobbing.

Always calm and observant, she would sit in the middle of the living room, serene and quiet as I ran around the room, a four-and-a-half-year-old doing cartwheels, turning somersaults, singing show tunes, kicking up my heels—anything to get attention and applause. At three-years-old, she already knew she was loved, she was enough, and didn't have to work for it.

She had a pretty singing voice, though she didn't think so. I taught her songs so we could sing harmony. We put on shows in the garage, big productions with make-up and costumes gleaned from my mother's cast-offs. In the backyard, we would perform acrobatic feats of wonder using the garden hose and creating a circus for all the neighborhood kids. We were a team—we were sisters.

We discovered books together and became bookworms, each checking out fourteen books a week from the local library, and reading all twenty-eight before they were returned and exchanged for a new tower of fourteen each. We worked through Mary Poppins, Little Women, Jack London and all the Oz books, the Shoes books (Ballet Shoes, Skating Shoes, etc.) and A Wrinkle in Time. We loved fantasy and stories about girls who were heroes.

Neither one was popular in high school; we were both smart, and fell into the Geeks and Hippies segment of the teen-age caste system. Bored with normal activities, we opened our own fashion boutique at fifteen and thirteen, designed and sewed all our own clothes, and with the help of our friends, we filled a whole store with our creations. We even made costumes for rock groups.

College for me, Europe for her. Then we came together again in the early 70's to open a Bikini Shop. We could do anything; we were sisters, and a team.

Relationships and marriages followed, years of working in the theater for me, years of working in publishing for her. We were always connected, always close.

Then, I was diagnosed with breast cancer, and she dropped everything to come and be with me and help. She cooked hundreds of meals and froze them, cleaned our house, top to bottom, and went with me to scary chemotherapy treatments. At forty-eight-years old, I finally learned what she had always known: that I was loved, I was enough; I didn't have to work for it.

I'm fine now, and she and I talk every week from 3,000 miles away. We're a deeply connected team, and our husbands joke about how lucky they are to have married the Olsen Sisters.

How could she be fifty? How could I be almost fifty-two? Well, that's the magic; she is really still my baby, and we're still singing songs together, putting on puppet shows in the garage, reading books and traveling the world. Every time I think of her, whether we are together or apart, we are all these things. She has been there with me, through all of it. We know all the secrets...we were there. Together.

I threw a big party for her fiftieth birthday. Everyone was asked to bring a skit or poem or song. We learned the song

"Sisters" from the movie, White Christmas, and performed it at the party; at the end, the crowd applauded and someone yelled, "Do it again. We want to hear it again!" So we did. And I'm sure we'll do it again and again over the next fifty years. The Olsen Girls never quit.

We're a team, forever and ever.
We're survivors. We're sisters.

Wouldn't It Be Nice....

If we found a cure for cancer. I feel we are getting closer. Thanks to all the breast cancer organizations and fundraising activities, more money is being spent to research breast cancer, and they are finding new drugs, new treatments, and people are living longer.

Conclusion

We have reached the end of our journey together, I'm sure you'll agree with me that this journey has been far more than a physical adventure through breast cancer medical treatments. The journey through breast cancer becomes emotional at times, spiritual in surprising ways, and absolutely life changing. We are not the same as when we started, we are different people, and we have shared it all. As a breast cancer survivor, you're not ever really alone. There are so many of us who have taken this tough road and made it back to tell the tale. There are so many who will come after us.We are united by a shocking turn of events that shook our lives up and changed us to the core.

Thank you for picking up this copy of my book the *#1 Best Tools and Tips from the Trenches of Breast Cancer.* It is my sincere wish that it has helped you on your medical journey through breast cancer and that you will pass it on to others to help them.

If you have any tools or tips to share, or any terrific products you think I should know about, please visit me on the website 1BestTTT.com and contribute to the Bulletin Board I've started for just that reason. You can also email me at CS4BCSoul@aol.com.

Don't stop reading just because this is the end of the book, some of my favorite products appear on the following pages under Products We Love in the Appendix. Tons of great products for breast cancer survivors are being invented every day, things that we not around six years ago when I was first diagnosed. Check them out! And please, do keep in touch.

Survive and Thrive with Love,
Mary Olsen Kelly

Appendix

Inspired Products and Services for the Breast Cancer Survivor

As a survivor, I know how difficult it is for most breast cancer patients to find products and services that could potentially make a huge difference in their level of comfort during and after chemo and radiation treatments. In keeping with the spirit of this book I've included the most current information possible on available products for you. I've discovered some amazing inventions designed to help you and me as breast cancer patients and survivors. Oral health enhancers like saliva stimulators, toothpaste and mouthwash with little or no alcohol in them; forward-thinking companies that make useful yet fashionable hospital gowns and yoga wear. I had no idea there were so many useful products out there, designed just for us.

Survivor Entrepreneurs

Every single one of us who goes through breast cancer face difficulties and challenges. Many of us want to "give back" in some way after our treatments are finished. The entrepreneurial survivors listed below were able to turn adversity into opportunity. As you'll discover, their efforts have resulted in a new vision, a new life and a new company. Here are women who were so challenged by the lack of services and comfort they encountered on their own medical journey that they invented solutions! These women, who saw a need and filled it, inspire me. Let me introduce you to them:

Healing Threads

Three sisters who created Healing Threads are determined to show that a person affected by breast cancer or any other disease can remain dignified, attractive, and comfortable while undergoing treatments. They invented a hospital jacket that is fashionable and functional. The Original Healing Threads is a soft cozy garment that insures your privacy. Each garment is equipped with such features as break away pieces that Velcro open and shut, to allow access during radiation treatments, or to ports for chemotherapy. Attractive enough to wear on the street, these beautiful garments insure that your dignity and privacy are respected.

Healing Threads
Spirited Sisters, Inc.
www.spirited-sisters.com
(877) 647-3900

Lumpectomy and Mastectomy Prosthesis and Bras

It took me five years to learn that there were prosthesis and bras for lumpectomy as well as mastectomy patients. I still can't believe that I walked around for five years with a size D cup on one side and a size B cup on the other. I felt embarrassed by the difference in size, and was painfully aware of the way the nipples hung at different heights. My clothes didn't fit well, and I developed a nagging "stitch" in my back—a little pain that never went away. Since I discovered the following companies and the fabulous bras and garments they provide, my life has changed for the better. Survivors started both companies, and they are filling a much-needed service to all of us.

Jodee

One great company for lumpectomy and mastectomy bras and prostheses in all sizes is Jodee. I have tried several of their bras and they are terrific. I am standing up straighter and looking better in my clothes. Best of all, that stitch in my back is gone!

"Jodee" Prosthesis and Bras
3100 North 29th Ave.
Hollywood, FLA 33020
(800) 423-9038

Still You

Another inspiring company is "Still You." I was so excited by my meeting with Heather Kuzmier, the owner and designer for "Still You," that I asked her to write a story for this book. She is enthusiastic, gorgeous, and filled with the passion of sharing her beautiful designs, a great example of a survivor who wants to help others. "Still You" is committed to making you feel that you're still beautiful after mastectomy. Yoga wear, athletic tanks, and camisoles with lightweight prosthesis are only a few of the items created by talented fashion designers at "Still You." Her designs are so popular that they are currently available in over two hundred breast boutiques nationwide.

Here's Heather's story:

Still You

Breast Cancer is a journey; often it is the turning tide that will lead you to do better, greater things with your life. Breast Cancer has had a very positive impact on my life. While going through lumpectomy, subsequent mastectomy and chemo, there were many things I felt were missing. Why could I not find something attractive and beautiful to wear? Why did I have to use a piece of something like quilting batting to replace my breast after surgery?

My mother-in-law sent my sister, my friend Carole and I to New York where we visited mastectomy boutiques looking for beautiful nightgowns. I so wanted to be beautiful, and feel beautiful after my mastectomy. We could not find anything that did not look like a grandmother's gown. I was disappointed and I clearly remember sitting in the cab next to my friend, Carole and saying, "We need to do something about this."

After surgery, I was given a polyester fluff ball to wear as a breast (for the first eight weeks) and a granny top to put it in. I was told to pull out some of the stuffing to get it to the right size. I felt that this was such an insult to a woman who had just given up a breast. Again, I told my friend Carole that we must do something about this.

During my chemotherapy we started testing new ideas. We developed a prosthesis, the first one that looked realistic, could be worn immediately after surgery and could also be used for swimming. We also started a line of fashionable contemporary clothing with bilateral bra pockets.

It is often said that cancer changes you. It is true. Cancer changes you in ways that you can never imagine. It is truly the most significant experience in my life because it led me to do something helpful and worthwhile for society. It caused me to refocus my life on my family and friends and things that truly matter.

"So many women say that they want to make a change and develop products for breast cancer, but few actually do," my physician said.

In less than one year after my surgery, we started our company: "Still You." At Still You, we recognize that each woman wants, needs, and deserves to look and feel beautiful. We are committed to providing women with an exceptional line of clothing to enhance self-esteem, build confidence and reflect the uniqueness of each woman. Our motto is: Still Confident, Still Beautiful, Still You.

—Heather Kuzmier
hkuzmier@StillYoufashions.com
Still You
www.stillyoufashions.com
(336) 282-9816

Personal Appearance

Make-up and beauty products can greatly enhance the way you feel about yourself during chemotherapy and radiation. Here is a great book, and a wonderful free service to help us feel and look better.

Facing the Mirror with Cancer
by Lori Ovitz
Julie@facingthemirror.org
(312) 214-3545

A beautiful book that teaches you to use make up to improve your appearance during cancer treatments.

If you are a breast cancer patient, you are eligible for free make up, wigs, scarves and training in how to use these items. Call your local American Cancer Society to find out when the next meeting is in your town. This is a wonderful free, non-medical program offered in partnership with the American Cancer Society, the National Cosmetology Assn. and the CTFA, a charitable organization supported by the cosmetic industry.

Look Good…Feel Better
www.lookgoodfeelbetter.com
(800) 395-LOOK

Women's Health Boutique

Vicki Dortch Jones and her sister, Seleta Dortch Lovell, founded Women's Health Boutique, "because women deserve more attention to their special needs."

Their mother, Billie Dortch, was diagnosed with terminal cancer in 1986. They were frustrated, wanting to make their mother's daily life easier and help restore her dignity that the cancer had taken away. It was only after Billie's death that the sisters were amazed to find so many products that could have helped her, that could have made her life more comfortable and that could restore a woman's dignity.

The mission of Women's Health Boutique is simple: "To meet women's special needs and make a positive difference in the way women look and feel about themselves. We are committed to excellence through compassion."

Women's Health Boutique offers a comfortable, dignified and discreet alternative to shopping for health-related merchandise—where personal service is the number one priority. Each of the beautiful Boutiques provides a relaxed setting where you will feel secure and at ease while selecting personal and intimate health care products. Fittings are done in private rooms with a certified fitter.

Women's Health Boutique
888.708.9982.
http://www.w-h-b.com/

Lifestyle Enhancers

The following products were extremely beneficial for me as I went through my treatments. Many of them are mentioned earlier as tips, but here is contact information.

It is hard to drink water during some phases of medical treatment.

Sobe drinks were delicious and easy to drink when I couldn't tolerate water. "Sobe" Drinks (especially Orange Carrot and Pink Grapefruit)

South Beach Beverages
Norwalk, CT
SoBeBev.Com

Tupperware is a company most of us remember from our childhood. They manufacture freezer containers in all sizes. They also make a Popsicle mold that can be used to make Chemo Pops .

"Tupperware" Popsicle Molds
Tupperware.com

One of the best and most soothing natural products for radiation burns comes straight from the **Aloe Vera** plant. The pure Aloe Vera gel can be found in most health food stores.

Aloe Vera Gel
For Radiation Burns
Available at Health Food Stores

Enjoy the benefits of drinking green and white tea. They are extremely good for fighting cancer and improving our immune system. Here's one of my favorite brands:

Republic of Tea
Green and White Tea
Novato, CA 94949
1-800-298-4TEA

I switched to natural grooming products wherever possible. I like this brand, "Tom's of Maine", a lot. The products are natural, they are available in most health food stores, and on the web.Tom's Toothpaste, Mouthwash, Deodorant

Tom's of Maine
P.O. Box 710
Kennebunk, ME 04043
www.TomsofMaine.com
1-800-FOR-TOMS

The Future Looks Bright

As a breast cancer survivor, I have a deep interest in new discoveries, new treatments and clinical trials, and new break-throughs toward finding a cure for breast cancer. We survivors hope and pray for a cure so that our daughters and granddaughters will not have to go through what we did.

I am not a medical professional, but as a breast cancer survivor I'm impressed with these new drugs and treatments. They give me hope and inspiration. Here are some that you might be interested in checking out.

Arimidex

I am finishing up five years of daily medication with Tomoxifan and getting ready to switch to Arimidex for several more years. The clinical trials have been so encouraging for Arimidex that I am really looking forward to taking it. If it can improve my life span I will be a big supporter!

Astra Zeneca
ARIMIDEX
P.O. Box 15437
Wilmington, DE 19850-5437
(800) 456-3669AstraZeneca.com

Herceptin

Some of the most exciting research is going on with the drug Herceptin. After tests and clinical trails, it looks like Herceptin will be available soon to be used by early stage breast cancer patients as well as those with metastases.

HERCEPTIN (trastuzmab)
Ganentech, Inc.
1 DNA Way
So. San Francisco, CA 94080
www.gene.com

Emla

One of the most helpful products during my medical journey with breast cancer was Emla numbing cream. I am a big fan of anything that minimizes pain and makes getting injections easier. Emla really saved me, I am so grateful that my friend Pandora told my sister about it, and that my sister asked the nurses to use it on me. Now I don't faint when I have blood drawn. This, for me, was a miracle.

EMLA
Astra Pharmaceuticals, L.P.
725 Chesterbrook Blvd.
Wayne, PA 19087-5677

Pain Ease Numbing Spray

Recently I have discovered other numbing agents similar to Emla. This is a terrific idea, a numbing spray. Pain Ease works in seconds to numb the skin for up to one minute. It is a spray that can be reapplied as needed. Like Emla, it is a topical numbing agent. Easy to use and fast, see if you don't think this is a winner.

Pain Ease
Gebauer Company
www.gebauerco.com
(800) 321-9348

Anti-Nausea

I would particularly like to thank the makers of Zofran because I know it was this drug that kept me from being nauseated during my chemotherapy. It helped me tremendously, and I shudder to think what my experience might have been without this terrific anti-nausea drug.

ZOFRAN (Ondansetron)
GlaxoSmithKline
1600 Vine St.

Philadelphia, PA 19102
www.gsk.com
(800) 366-8900

More Anti-Nausea

Any type of anti-nausea drug is a good idea in my opinion. Emend is another type of drug that offers a similar result, no nausea! Hooray!

EMEND
Merck and Co., Inc.
351 N. Sumneytown Pike
North Wales, PA 19454
www.merck.com

Neupogen

When my white blood cell count dropped after each chemotherapy treatment, my husband Don did a great job of injecting me with a syringe of Neupogen every day for nine days following treatment. This wonderful drug boosted my cell production, making it possible for me to stay on schedule and be strong enough for my next round of chemo. I called Don "Dr. Feelgood!"

NEUPOGEN (filgrastim)
Amgen Inc. One Amgen Center Drive
Thousand Oaks, CA 91320
www.amgen.com

Xylocaine Mouthwash Gel

Lidocaine (Xylocaine) A local anesthetic that is effective, safe, and reliable topical wash or mouthwash antiseptic.

Prescribed by doctor
www.Drugstore.com

Biotene

Medications, radiation, illness, or normal aging can cause dry mouth. Daily use of Biotene's effective bio-active enzymatic therapy helps reduce the symptoms of Dry Mouth and helps relieve bleeding gums, gingivitis, minor gum irritations, and harmful bacteria.

Biotene Dry Mouth Toothpaste
Prescribed by doctor
www.laclede.com

Prevention Oncology Mouth Rinse

This mouth rinse contains only 1.6% alcohol and is clinically proven to heal ulcerations and preserve the normal, healthy bacteria while killing the rest. The low alcohol content makes it easier on your mouth during chemo. Sold over the counter at most drug stores and Walmart.

www.Preventionmouthrinse.com
(800) 473-1205

Soothing Mouth Care

A range of oral care products including Gel Toothpaste, Saliva Substitute, Mouth Rinse, Lip Moisturizer and others designed to sooth delicate oral tissue and prevent dry mouth.

Soothing Mouth Care Gel
Moisturizer Saliva Substitute
Tri-State Hospital Supply
(800) 248-4058

Drain Management

This looks like an excellent new dressing for port/catheter site management. The transparent "window" shaped bandage has an integrated pad that wicks moisture away and provides a strong barrier against bacteria. It is latex-free and hypo-allergenic. It manages multiple drain tubes while giving continuous site visibility.

SorbaView
2000 Window Dressing
www.tshsc.com
(800) 248-4058

Medical Communities that Care

As a breast cancer patient, we are never really alone. Behind us, stand thousands of support people; families, friends, co-workers, nurses, doctors, scientists, drug manufacturers, hospital personnel, product designers and suppliers. The list goes on and on.

It takes a special kind of person to go into the field of nursing, and the most dedicated nurses of all are those that specialize in oncology (cancer). I have never met such warm, sincere, and genuinely caring people in my life. I want to extend my heartfelt thanks to all the dedicated professionals who work tirelessly to bring hope and inspiration to those of us with breast cancer.

There are doctors all over the country who really are true healers; there are surgeons who specialize only in breast surgery. To these caring professionals, I extend a bouquet of pink ribbons from all the millions of breast cancer survivors you have saved.

Throughout the United States, there are hospitals with Breast Centers, Cancer Centers, Women's Health Boutiques, Quality of Life Centers, and Wellness Centers integrated right into the hospitals. In many of these hospitals there are Nurse Navigators who guide the newly diagnosed breast cancer patient through a medical maze. Thank you with all our hearts for continually improving the environment and the services for those newly-diagnosed as well as long term survivors.

When you think about it, there are actually millions of people all working hard for the benefit of breast cancer patients and survivors. How many millions run the Race for the Cure every year? How many thousands do the Three Day Walk for the Cure in cities all over the country? The quantity of support for us is mind-boggeling!

We even have our own month; October is Breast Cancer Awareness month. How many people can boast that they have their very own month? I want to thank everyone who has been touched by breast cancer, all the families and friends, all the husbands and lovers, all the children who have helped Mommy get well. Without families and friends, the journey would not be successful. Thank you to everyone who buys a breast cancer stamp and uses it to mail a letter, just to benefit all of us breast cancer survivors.

Let's give a standing ovation to the pink ribbon ladies who raise millions of dollars for breast cancer research, all the walkers and runners and fund-raisers who have made this a top priority. Because of you, there is much more money available for research and improvements. Thanks to all of you, we are in the Pink! Because of your love, care, support, and professional abilities, we can and we do survive and thrive!

And last but not least, I send love, light, health and sunshine to breast cancer survivors everywhere. We have fought a fierce battle and won to celebrate another day, and another year, and another decade. We are heroes, who deserve to live our lives filled with love, health and happiness. Together we transform our challenges into pearls of strength, healing, and fruitful and fulfilling lives.

Thank you, one and all.

Resources

American Cancer Society
National Call Center
1599 Clifton Road NE
Atlanta, GA 30329-4251
(800) ACS-2345
www.cancer.org

General Information, education and support services including Reach to Recovery, Look Good-Feel Better, Making Strides, and other ACS programs.
www.lookgoodfeelbetter.org

MAMM Magazine
54 West 22nd Street, 4th floor
New York, NY 10010
www.Mamm.com

Mamm is an excellent resource. It is a magazine just for breast cancer and ovarian cancer survivors. Every issue is filled with the latest news in the medical field, and has wonderful articles by and for survivors.

The Susan G. Komen Breast Cancer Foundation
5005 LBJ Freeway, Suite 370
Dallas, TX 75244
www.Komen.org

Volunteers work through local chapters and Race for the Cure events to further the Foundation's mission of eradicating breast cancer as a life-threatening disease by advancing research, education, screening, and treatment. Trained caring volunteers answer national toll free helpline. (800) I'M AWARE 462-9273

National Alliance of Breast Cancer Organizations
9 East 37th St.
NY, NY 10016
(800) 719-9154 or (212) 889-0606
www.nabco.org

A network of Breast Cancer organizations that provides information, education, assistance, and referral to anyone with questions about breast cancer, and acts as a voice for the interests and concerns of breast cancer survivors and women at risk. The NABREAST CANCERO resource list is a very comprehensive and available for a small fee or with membership.

Kids Konnected
(800) 899-2866
www.kidskonnected.org

A hotline Internet site and support group for kids to talk to other kids.

KidsCope
(404) 892-1437
www.kidscope.org

Educational materials to help kids cope when a family member has cancer.

Kid Support
(847) 869-1323
www.kid-support.org

Adult-led peer-support counseling for kids.

Cancer Information Service
(800) 4 CANCER
www.cancer.gov

Part of the National Cancer Institute, offering free publications or the opportunity to talk directly to cancer specialists on treatment and prevention of cancer. Also available in Spanish.

The Mautner Project for Lesbians with Cancer
(202) 332-5536
www.mautnerproject.org

Offers education and information for lesbians with cancer, their partners and families.

National Breast Cancer Coalition
1707 L. Street NW Suite 1060
Washington, DC 20036
(202) 296-7477
www.natlbcc.org

A grassroots advocacy group that trains and activates all women and men concerned about this disease to effectively focus the public, scientific community, Congress, and the Administration on increasing funding into the causes and cure for breast cancer, improving women's access to high quality care, and increasing the involvement and influence of women with breast cancer in setting policy.

National Cancer Institute Cancer Information Service
(800) 4 cancer
http://www.cancer.gov

A hot line with up to date information on cancer for patients and families, as well as the general public.

Wellness Community
(888) 793-WELL
www.thewellnesscommunity.org

Provides free emotional and psychological support to cancer patients and their children 5-18.
(888) 793-WELL
www.thewellnesscommunity.org

Y-Me
212 W. Van Buren, 4th flr
Chicago, IL 60607
(800) 221-2141
(800) 986-9505 - Spanish
www.y-me.org

Provides information, education, counseling, and free wigs and prosthesis for women with financial need. Will ship for a small handling fee. A national hotline is available 24-7.

Revlon/UCLA Women's Cancer Research Program
Known for the celebrity-studded annual fund-raiser the "Fire and Ice Ball," Revlon/UCLA Women's Cancer Research Program serves women with a combination of research, treatment and outreach programs. "This program is altering the course of medicine," asserted Lilly Tartikoff, who founded the program in 1990 with Ronald Perelman, chairman of Revlon, and UCLA's Dr. Dennis Slamon.

Breast Cancer.Org
Breastcancer.org, a web-based nonprofit organization providing around the clock expert medical information and support, has been recognized for the second consecutive year as a leader among the 1,200 web sites entered in the annual eHealthcare Leadership Awards. See pictures of TRAM Flap,

Tissue Expanders, Latissimus Dorsi Flap Reconstruction, and more. Dr. Marisa C. Weiss, founder of Breastcancer.org, is a practicing oncologist.

Suggested Reading

Newly Diagnosed and Treatment Survival:

The Breast Cancer Book of Strength and Courage; Inspiring Stories to See You Through Your Journey by Ernie Bodai, M.D., F.A.C.S. and Judie Fertig Panneton, Prima Publishing.

This book is all stories from survivors. There are forty-six stories, many of them very long. The book is excellent; it is inspiring and acts as proof that a book of this type is powerfully effective in lifting the spirits of survivors.

Chicken Soup for the Breast Cancer Survivor's Soul; Stories to Refresh the Soul and Rekindle the Spirit by Jack Canfield, Mark Victor Hansen, and Mary Olsen Kelly, HCI Publishing.

A collection of heart-warming, inspirational stories from breast cancer survivors, this is an excellent book. It is a "support group between two covers" that shares lots of information and memorable stories, some funny, some sad. This book lets the reader know that she is not alone.

Living Beyond Breast Cancer; A Survivors Guide For When Treatment Ends and the Rest of Your Life Begins by Marisa C. Weiss, M.D., and Ellen Weiss, Times Books, Random House.

This is an excellent book to read after all your treatments and surgery are completed and you are trying to get on with your life. It covers everything from medical concerns, managing your ongoing health care with your team of specialists, to emotional, sexual, career and self-esteem issues. Written by a doctor who specializes in breast cancer, this book is an excellent resource.

Medical:

Dr. Susan Love's Breast Book by Susan M. Love, MD with Karen Lindsey, De Capo Press.

This book is the essential guide to understanding your medical pathology written by a breast specialist. This is the bible of breast cancer, it explains everything about cancer, surgery, chemotherapy, radiation, from a doctor's point of view. This is the best medical book on breast cancer, in my opinion.

Love, Medicine and Miracles by Bernie Siegel, M.D. Harper and Row;

Peace, Love and Healing by Bernie Siegel, M.D., Harper and Row.

Dr. Bernie Siegel is famous for his revolutionary work pioneering the body-mind connection in the arena of western medicine. He shares his experience as a surgeon, working with what he calls "Exceptional Patients," those that survive far longer than expected. Dr. Siegel shares the attitudes and behaviors of those patients, and analyses why he thinks that they live longer. These two books are wonderful, both offer the reader many ways to utilize the tools and techniques for self-healing.

Getting Well Again by O. Carl Simonton M.D., Stephanie Matthews-Simonton, and James L. Creighton, Bantam Books.

This best-selling classic shares self-awareness, mind-body connection, and self-healing techniques. Dr. Simonton is known as the father of psychoneuroimmunology, psychosocial medicine, an approach that combines medical and psychological techniques in the treatment of cancer. The Simontons are credited with the first use of visualization, such as imagining little pac-mans eating cancer cells, in the treatment of cancer.

For Children:

Our Family Has Cancer, Too by Christine Clifford, University of Minnesota Press.

The Year My Mother Was Bald by Ann Speltz, Magination Press

Sammy's Mommy Has Cancer by Sherry Kohlenberg, Magination Press

Spiritual:

Close to the Bone; Life Threatening Illness and the Search for Meaning by Jean Shinoda Bolen, M.D., Simon & Schuster, Inc.

In this beautifully written book, the author explores the way serious illness brings us close to the bone, close to our soul. Using the powerful imagery of myth, she explores the connection between illness and the heroic journey. Innana, Persophone, Psyche, and other goddesses from mythology give hope and guidance to the reader under Dr. Bolen's skilled hand.

When Bad Things Happen to Good People by Harold S. Kushner, Harper, Collins Publishers.

Excellent book offers and humane and moving approach to inexplicable illness. For all of us who must contend with suffering, this book will make you feel better. Written by a Rabbi, and exploring the spiritual aspects of pain, hardship, and disease, this best selling book has brought peace to millions.

Art. Rage.Us. Art and Writing by Women with Breast Cancer, introduction by Jill Eikenberry, epilogue by Terry Tempest Williams, Chronicle Books.

This collection of art works by over seventy artists is so stunning, moving and powerful that I have included it in the spiritual category. The combination of art and outrage was originally exhibited in San Francisco to bring attention to breast cancer. The book is a must read for all survivors.

The Best Personal Stories:

The Victoria's Secret Catalog Never Stops Coming and other lessons I learnedfrom Breast Cancer, by Jennie Nash, Penguin Putnam, Inc.

Author Jennie Nash is a wonderful storyteller. Her heartwarming tales of family and the small incidents of life are moving and inspiring. This is a great book.

It's Not About The Bike; My Journey Back to Life, by Lance Armstrong, Penguin Putnam, Inc.

Few people are as inspiring as Lance Armstrong. This book details his journey through cancer and recovery and it is a powerful motivational story. He went through hell, and went on to win the Tour de France—again!

The Best Alternative Healing Books:

Instant Healing, *by Serge Kahili King,* Renaissance Publishing.

This is a wonderful book filled with healing techniques that really work. Highly recommended, along with all of Dr. Kings other books: Urban Shaman, Huna Healing, etc.

You Can Heal Your Life by Louise Hay, Hay House.

This is a classic in the field of healing and consciousness. Louise Hay healed herself of cancer using the techniques shared in this useful book.

Creative Visualization, by Shakti Gawain, New World Library.

Nutrition:

Eat to Beat Cancer, by J. Robert Hatherhill, Ph.D., Renaissance Books.

The Cancer Lifeline Cookbook, by Kimberly Mathai, M.S., R.D., with Ginny Smith, Sasquatch Books.

Eating Well Through Cancer, by Holly Clegg and Gerald Miletello, M.D., Wimmer Cookbooks.

Special terms available direct from the Publisher

If you or your organization is interested in purchasing quantities of *#1 Best Tools and Tips from the Trenches of Breast Cancer* for fund raising or promotion, please contact:

Barbara Curtis—Publisher
Books Beyond Borders LLC
P.O. Box 18696
South Lake Tahoe, CA 96151
Fax (916) 541-6021
email curtisbbb@charter.net
Or visit our website
www.1bestTTT.com

#1 Best Tools and Tips from the Trenches of Breast Cancer is also available for purchase from Amazon.com, Barnes & Noble, Justbookz.com, and through Ingram as well as fine bookstores everywhere.

Praise for Mary Olsen Kelly's *Path of the Pearl:*

"*Path of the Pearl* offers new ways to face the hardest challenges of life and transform them into opportunities for creating beauty, love, and power."

> —**Susan Jeffers, Ph.D.,** Author of *Feel the Fear and Do It Anyway* and *End the Struggle and Dance with Life.*

"This book is a poetic journey of self-love combined with powerful tools and techniques for transforming life's challenges into creations of beauty."

> —**Jack Canfield,** CO-creator #1 NY Times Best-selling series *Chicken Soup for the Soul.*

"Art from adversity. Beauty from irritation. Like the pearl, our inner growth develops as we accept and adapt to the unexpected. This beautiful book is a gracious guide to nurturing ourselves on the very deepest levels."

> —**Diana von Welenetz Wentworth,** co-author with Jack Canfield and Mark Victor Hansen of *Chicken Soup for the Soul Cook Book* and the romantic memoir *Send Me Someone.*